The Floater's Log

A Book
By
Ronald Krome

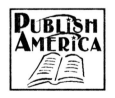

PublishAmerica
Baltimore

ISBN: 1-4241-8282-4
PUBLISHED BY PUBLISHAMERICA, LLLP
www.publishamerica.com
Baltimore

Printed in the United States of America

DEDICATION

This book is dedicated to the men and women who served as floaters, and whose commitment to receiving and the citizens of Detroit are unequaled. And to:

Charles Krome	Gerald Mailloux
Eva Mae Krome	Mary Lamont
Morris Kanow	William Mailloux
Sol Koren	Nancy Simpson
Freida Bulmash	

And to all those who contributed to my career and mostly my life, whether living or dead

They are immortal in my heart.

Do not stand by my grave and weep
I am not there. I do not sleep.
I am a thousand winds that blow.
I am the diamond's glint on snow.
I am the sunlight and ripened grain.
I am the gentle autumn rain.
When you awake in the morning hush,
I am the swift uplifting rush of quiet birds in circling flight.
I am the soft starlight at night.
Do not stand by my grave and weep.
I am not there. I do not sleep.

—Anonymous

Dedicated also to my sons, Charles, Jonathan, Christopher and Brian, and to my daughters, Amy Beth and Janette; and to my wife, Marcy, without whose help, loyalty and love I couldn't have done this project.

Chapter I
Prelude

What I have recorded here, in a semi-narrative fashion, are the events surrounding my tenure as an emergency physician and chief of emergency medicine at Detroit Receiving Hospital from 1969 through 1984. For me it was a time of growing up and becoming an adult man. Be that as it may, recorded are the comments of various other physicians, all of which will be explained, in italics. I did not change their words or correct their English or grammar, even if it would have made better reading. Rather I left it as entered in the Floater's Log, so it would be more realistic.

In reality, my journey began nine years earlier, when I made a ten-day road trip looking for an internship. These were the days when no intern matching process existed, one had to seek out and negotiate for the opportunity.

I was born and raised in Baltimore, Maryland, and had married while in medical school. I had two objectives for my trip. Accompanied by wife, I was looking for a unique training setting in a community we could live. The hospitals on the East Coast paid little or nothing for interns. I remember when Johns Hopkins was forced to begin paying their house officers. It was considered an honor for medical students to go there for training. In one of my interviews, my interviewer even said this.

So when we got back to Baltimore, we decided to go Detroit for training at Detroit's Receiving Hospital, where I stayed for virtually my entire professional life. The hospital paid well for that time—three hundred dollars per month—had a great staff and was a "doing" hospital—someplace where the residents carried the load and did virtually everything.

We found an apartment on the west side of the city, settled in, and began living. I began my internship, and, as a matter of fact, was on rounds on gynecology when I received an overhead page—there were no beepers then—I tried to ignore it but my intern colleagues insisted. When I answered, the operator told me there was an accident and my wife was at Mt. Carmel Hospital. I called and was told to come to the ER right away. My wife had been in a serious accident and they couldn't tell me anything else.

I borrowed a car and was at Carmel in record time. I went into the ER, taken to private room, and told to wait. Shortly, a resident showed up, brushing food particles from his mouth, and told me my wife was dead. I couldn't believe it. I told him he had made a mistake. He said nothing but took me to a body on a gurney. It was Eva; cold, dead.

I stood holding the hand and kissing my once vivacious, warm and gregarious wife, when suddenly one of my intern colleagues showed up. This was August, and we hardly knew each another. The operator at Receiving had told him what happened. He came to help. To be honest, I couldn't have gotten through the next several weeks without him.

I remain unsure of what prepared me to take this job. I know I was ready. As Pasteur once said, "Chance favors the prepared mind." But there were things that helped me mature and get ready.

Certainly the five-year surgical residency I had just completed was a big factor in my growth and development. This was what was called, in those days, a "cutting residency." Although there were a lot of faculty and senior resident supervision, everyone operated, from your first year through their last.

One of the most maturing events in the residency was the "M&M (Mortality & Morbidity) Conference." This was a mandatory conference for residents, almost always run by the Chairman, or another senior faculty member. At this conference any death in the hospital, wherever it occurred, while the patient was on the surgical service, or any complication of surgery, was presented by the operating surgeon, meaning the surgical resident. Although some time was spent discussing the operation or the patient's disease, the bulk of the time was in discussion of what could have been done differently to prevent the complication or patient death. The assumption was always that the operating surgeon was responsible for the adverse event (isn't that a great euphemism!).

It was here that the resident stood up and took his licks. It was hard on almost all of us. Sometimes residents cried. But they all paid their *mea culpa.* Here is where you grew up and became an adult. But there were tricks to getting through it without being scalped.

In the early days, I really had trouble learning how to come out of the conference intact. Finally, one of the junior faculty took pity on me. He told me that when I present, I should present the case, and then list the errors I made. Not leave any out; that way, no one can say that I did anything wrong. I had already admitted them. Things went much better for me after that.

It was a hard residency and you had to work hard and long to get through it. There was no limit on the hours that you had to spend at the hospital. And when you were a senior resident you were on call at all times, and had to come in whenever necessary. On one of my rotations, the Chief's Service, I had filled the ICU with my patients, and even had several in the Recovery Room. The isolation room in Recovery was called by the nurses the "Krome Room." I spent ten consecutive days and nights in the hospital, sometimes coming home for dinner and going right back, sleeping there. The Chief made rounds with me, but mostly I had to work things out for myself.

I had one patient who had sustained a gunshot of the abdomen, injuring five separate organs. He made it through the operation well. We had done things by the book and he was in ICU. I went over him the next day with the Chief. I was so proud and so excited by the outcome that my enthusiasm was bubbling over. When rounds were

7

over the Chief took me on the side. "Ron," he said, "I can see how pleased you are at the outcome of this patient. And I believe it is justified. But this patient will die in five to seven days, and there is nothing you can do to prevent it." I was crushed, and thought, no way. He was dead in five days—sepsis; kidney failure; heart failure; and finally, multiple organ failure. Needless to say I was crushed. I couldn't believe it. My whole team had spent five days and nights working to save him.

I worked the Detroit riots (civil disturbance?) all five days. On the first night, I was called at home by a surgical attending who said that something was going on and I should keep myself available. While I was talking to him, I turned on the television and watched the havoc starting. I told him if I was needed, decide now, because I wouldn't come in until everything was over, if I didn't come in now. So I went in and spent five days and nights at the hospital. I shared my on call room with two National Guard. I worked Triage and was on one of the surgical teams. We worked twelve hours on and eight off. The eight quickly went away. All the rioters who came in had swollen jaws and gastroenteritis. There were a lot of fractured jaws.

There was one soldier who came in with a large dental abscess and fever. His tooth was pulled and he immediately went back to work. The soilders who came in had just came back from Vietnam and weren't happy at all. When they left to go on patrol, they would tell us that we would not receive any injured rioters. They would take care of it. We had more DOA's than reported in the media!

On the night my appointment was announced, about two in the morning, the phone rang: "You're out of your fucking mind!" I was home in bed. .

It was 1969 and I just finished my surgical residency at Detroit Receiving Hospital — and accepted a position on the hospital's surgical staff with orders to "straighten out the emergency room." The surgery chief hired me, and described it as a "unique challenge." Emergency medicine wasn't a recognized medical specialty, and ERs (emergency rooms) were a far cry from that seen nowadays. There was, at that time, no recognition of emergency medicine; so there was little hope of making progress in the academic world.

Not everyone thought I was making a wise career decision, to say the least. The interesting thing was that the man, who called me, later went to work in emergency medicine.

Young faculty assigned to the emergency room, as I was, across the country represented a wide variety of specialties. As soon as feasible, most left emergency medicine and returned to their original field. Few if any, continued in emergency medicine. I did.

I loved working in the emergency room, something I had done quite a bit of during my residency. I liked, and like, the action; the quick decision making necessary; and the variety of medical problems faced daily, from major trauma to minor illnesses, liked the fact that the emergency room was the center of the hospital and the conscience of the community. This large emergency room was surrounded by a relatively small hospital. It was the center of action.

I liked feeling needed by the community, not just the patients. I was, and am, proud of our commitment to them. The emergency room was where the start of epidemics was identified and where social problems were addressed, and when people had no place else to go, they came to the emergency room. We are and have remained the safety net. Working there certainly gave me an adrenaline rush.

In 1961, when I arrived fresh out of medical school, Receiving already had a forty year history of serving the poor. Its reputation as an emergency hospital was manifest before my arrival, and was contingent on it. Receiving started as a city owned hospital in downtown Detroit, dedicated to the masses. It was always poorly funded. The basis of its national and international reputation rested largely on the surgery department and trauma. The public considered it the place to go if critically ill or injured, otherwise you should stay away. A poor hospital poorly funded for poor people. Many of the physicians in Michigan came from Receiving and Wayne State University School of Medicine.

When I started and for sometime afterwards, the hospital was known as "Receiving." Although our colleagues at Wayne County General Hospital (the county's hospital), called us "Detroit Sending Hospital" because of the patients we sent them. I had selected this hospital for my internship because it offered a wide variety of pathology, good staff supervision, and an ability of the house officers to do "things;" it was a doing hospital, resident run.

To change our image, in 1972, the city decided to call us "Detroit General Hospital." It didn't work. Our patients didn't change; nor did our image. In 1980, as we were getting ready to move into the new hospital, a staff survey chose "Receiving" as the name.

We saw 100,000-150,000 patients each year, without regard to sex, sexual orientation, race or religion, or ability to pay. Laws mandating this didn't exist; we did it anyhow. Patients were transferred to us because they couldn't pay. Detroit was healing from the riots of 1967. Receiving, with a sixty-year history of providing care to all comers, was, for better or worse, like a MASH unit in the ongoing battle to bring the Motor City back to life.

Patients mostly didn't have insurance (Now, thanks to HMO's, we transfer them out when they do have it!) or were unemployed. Worse, for the patients, they often came unannounced meaning we had to start all over, delaying definitive treatment. Patients would be dumped off, sometimes near death, sometimes after it, at the rear entrance (the ambulance dock); especially when family and friends were involved and the patients were shot, stabbed, or drugged. Before abortions were legalized, many women, and girls, were transferred to us with septic abortions or severe vaginal bleeding. There were instances when they arrived with transfusions running. In their desire to terminate their pregnancy women would use coat hangers, pencils, pens and potassium permanganate douches.

Over the years, I noticed when patients got their own insurance, or got government coverage they stopped coming to us. It was as though the community itself thought we did not accept insurance. But when they lost it they came back. I think that patients and staff believed that we didn't accept patients with insurance. I overhead some staff, in fact, tell patients and relatives that we didn't accept insurance.

Transferred patients arrived mostly in private ambulances. Public ambulance services didn't exist. Trauma patients, picked up on the street, were brought in by the police, in station wagons, fast enough, but no IV's (intravenous fluids), oxygen, or backboards. The police bragged they could get to any of the city's thirty to forty ERs in less than five minutes—and delivered on those claims—but the lack of pre-hospital care would stun many of today's emergency medical personnel. Some patients arrived in private cars or taxis.

In 1972, Detroit formed its EMS (Emergency Medical Service), as a part of the DFD (Detroit Fire Department), a development stimulated by the death by a young girl—a death not in vain.

She had fallen out of a tree in Detroit's Belle Isle—a public park in the middle of the Detroit River, and lapsed quickly into unconsciousness. The police were called and quickly responded. She was placed in the back of a station wagon, on a fold up gurney (no oxygen, no neck precautions), and conveyed to the closest hospital, arriving in less than five minutes. .

The emergency entrance was locked so they had to ring a bell to summon staff. A nurse and an intern, he just two months out of medical school, informed the police that they had neither facilities nor personnel to handle this problem. The intern never examined the child. Everyone went back to the wagon, which wouldn't start (Murphy's Law). A second wagon was called and took everyone to Receiving, where they were met by a neurosurgical team.

She died in the operating room. A lawsuit and community uproar, both of which were justified, followed. The outcome was Detroit EMS. I don't know if the family ever realized what their daughter's death did for the city.

During my internship, the Chrysler Freeway was being built. There was a ditch and little else. I was working in the emergency room and the police brought in a young boy who had slid down the wall of the ditch to the valley below. On his way down he managed to impale himself on a piece of wooden fence. Of course, the police were called. They brought the boy in with the piece still in him. He was lying on his abdomen. Every time the car drove over a bump, the piece sticking out, about four feet of wood would bounce up and down. About one foot of fence stuck out above. There was about one foot in him. The larger piece was sawed off. He was lucky the piece in him never touched anything and went through his subcutaneous fat. It was removed without any problem.

In preparation for EMS, a survey of Detroit's thirty-five emergency rooms and hospitals was done in 1970. Many of the ER's were understaffed, and under equipped. The results, presented at a meeting of hospital representatives, were not met with great joy. Many at the meeting had even helped design the survey and conducted it. Those that yelled the loudest were from hospitals that failed to get a higher ranking than listed. Eventually, a list was provided EMS that contained the medical or trauma problems the hospital shouldn't get. I remain unsure why any hospital would want patients for whom they were unable to provide proper care. Evidently, they didn't want it known publicly they weren't full service.

Three hospitals closed their emergency business entirely. Detroit began its EMS. And the medical community began to realize the need for better ER care.

As a part of determining which agency would be given the responsibility of operating EMS, Wayne State University School of Medicine, using the staff of the emergency room, conducted a study. Three groups, similar in numbers and age, fire personnel, police, and private ambulance companies, were given training in first responder care. All were trained together at the same time. They were put on the street, and their ability to apply and willingness to use, their skills were measured. The fire fighting personnel far and away used and applied their skill most frequently; were most willing to help the sick and injured and apply their training. This really didn't surprise anyone, and it still shouldn't. The fire department has a multi-century tradition of helping. Not so for the others.

The units were put on the street, each manned by two EMT'S.

Before Detroiters were accustomed to EMS responding to 911 calls, a unit was dispatched to an apartment, knocked on the door, and went in when invited. The EMT's were met by a man with a shot gun aimed right at them.

What are you doing here?

You called because you are sick.

I thought the police would come. I want to get me a cop.

We'll get one for you.

When they turned to leave, one EMT opened a door and walked into a closet. Both managed to get out intact.

Even today many of the calls to 911 are not emergencies. People call for transportation to clinics, doctors' offices, or asking a variety of questions, not all related to healthcare.

Receiving was often filthy; except, of course, when it was being inspected or visited by a local politician. Because DRH was owned by the City of Detroit, under the health department, we were a popular destination for local politicians, especially before elections.

The only regular visitors were pests of another sort: flies and insects. No matter the elected officials and wannabes who came through never brought money. Without funding for either effective air conditioning or window screens, our insect friends couldn't wait to drop by during the hot Detroit summers, when the rooms were so stifling we had no choice but to open windows.

Fly paper strips were as common as IVs, but the bugs out maneuvered our defense. They were better organized, too. They were an integral part of the hospital routine and folklore. We had the "Q" sign, for comatose patients who had their tongues out of one corner of their mouths, making their faces look like "Q's," and indicating severe illness, but not necessarily death. To this, we added the "three fly" sign: any patient who allowed three or more flies to rest on their bodies at one time, without flinching or moving, had the "three fly" sign. Not many walked out.

"Frequent fliers" were a collection of patients and visitors that often came to visit, mostly for the entertainment value of the ER. They were a motley crew that came so often they were on a first-name basis with staff. An assortment of drunks, drug abusers, and people, who just couldn't afford medical care, and even some patients with insurance, would come often; some for the entertainment value, some for food and warmth. They came so often, and for so little, we labeled them, "ER groupys."

There were three groups of drinkers: (one) the angry drunks, who spoke with numerous expletives, often reflecting on our parentage — either the lack thereof or our incestuous relationships with same, especially our mothers. Threats of great bodily harm and major lawsuits were also part of the fun; (two) the quiet drunks who swore they were done drinking forever or at least for the next twenty-four hours; (three) the warm and friendly drunks, the con artists, inebriated or not, who had an ability to wheedle the nursing and medical staff out of food and blankets. Another way to group them was as angry drunks and not angry drunks. But no matter what category or group they were in, they all had the potential to become chronic alcoholics, drinking themselves into oblivion.

Many were looking for a place to flop and something to eat. If we weren't too busy, and sometimes even if we were, we accommodated them. The nurses would let them sleep it off and provide them with the same fare given to other patients: a piece of cheese between two slices of white bread, with perhaps some juice or milk. I still have one of those sandwiches, which I'm proud to say, became known as a "Kromeburger," bronzed and mounted on a plaque by a class of graduating residents. I imagine it tastes pretty much the same now, bronzed, as it did some thirty-five years ago! During the winter, the homeless slept outside on warm air vents or along covered walls. Some built houses of cardboard boxes, on the street, using newspapers as blankets.

Once, I found one frequent flyers, PF, sitting, at Triage, waiting to be seen. I told him we were too busy to attend to his scratched finger and too busy to get him a sandwich. He left, but he wasn't happy. I underestimated him enormously.

Two hours later, I found him in a treatment room, sitting on a gurney, eating a sandwich and drinking milk. PF had pulled a fire alarm. He waited for the fire department, admitted what he had done, and was arrested. The police promptly brought him to us, because he told them he had an infected cut on his finger! The nurses knew PF so well that when he died, they pitched in to pay for his burial. Sometime later, a small park with benches was built across the street from the hospital. It was dubbed the "PF Memorial Park."

PF went to that big saloon in the sky.

Entry in log: 4/1/77.

A happy drunk was wandering around the treatment room where I was working, wearing a nice three piece suit. He proudly let me know that when he died, he was going to donate his brain to science. A tempting offer, but I told him we didn't want it because it was pickled. He thought this was the funniest thing he ever heard, and walked through the entire ER letting everyone know his brain had been rejected by the medical establishment. I never saw him — or his brain — again.

After we were in the new hospital (DRH), two EMT's came in wheeling an obviously intoxicated man, in a wheelchair. Both EMT's were smiling as wide as they could. I could tell something was going on, so I stopped them. They handed me their run slip. Transfer from was DGH; to DRH. The patient was sleeping in my office at the old hospital (DGH). Continuity of care!

Staffing posed its own challenges. Just as much as DRH's ER was a dumping ground for patients, it was the same for staff. Nurses were often transferred there as punishment or because they couldn't function on the floors. Equipment was handed down from the operating room; frequently broken or on the edge of the trash bin. Until we could order our own, we were at the mercy of others. Respirators and suction units were ordered from central supply on an as needed basis.

One orderly showed a unique approach to patient care. One psychiatric patient made some disparaging remarks about the orderly's mother. Although the patient was "four-pointed" (all four limbs restrained), that didn't stop the orderly from beating him. Naturally, he was fired, although he couldn't understand why. After all, the patient had said some very nasty things about his mother. The orderly claimed it was self defense.

While this kind of behavior from staff was rare, the violent behavior of some patients was not. Once, when I was making rounds, an elderly woman, around the mid-'80s, asked to see whoever was supervising the doctors. She was restrained one arm and one leg. That was me. I came to her bedside and asked her what the problem was. Her response was to haul off and back hand me with her free arm with enough force to send me reeling, to the floor, and my glasses flying.

Residents (house officers) were assigned to the ER for some period of their training. Many didn't want to be there — and it showed. They essentially ran the ER, supervising junior residents and students, but without any supervision of their own. The first assistant surgical resident, known as the "pit boss," was responsible for making rounds and seeing every single patient, regardless of medical problem. In essence, this was a surgically run ER.

Mornings began with the pit boss and senior medical resident trying to wake the drunks. Those that couldn't be roused went to neurosurgery for a head injury consultation. Those with the DT's (delirium tremens=an alcohol withdrawal syndrome) were admitted. The death rate for patients with DT's was nearly thirty percent then. Patients with abdominal pain and/or tenderness, and vomiting, were checked for pancreatitis, an inflammation of the pancreas that often afflicts chronic alcoholics. "Healthy" frequent fliers left to go about their day's routine, usually sent off with an "I'll see you tonight" by the staff. To make sure they really left, the gurney mattresses were folded up and put under the gurney.

By the early '70s the number of house officers with English as a second language had begun to increase. DGH couldn't have survived without them.

Because there were so few attending physicians in the ER — and emergency residencies didn't exist at that time — manpower was a constant problem. We hired residents from other specialties to moonlight. They were poorly paid and without specific emergency experience or qualifications. The moonlighters were working the "dirty thirties," named for the thirty dollars an hour they were paid. There weren't even ACLS (Advanced Cardiac Life support) or ATLS (Advanced Trauma Life support) programs available.

The attendings who were there…well, there was one doctor who "worked" the ER when I took the job. I don't remember how long he had been there, how long he stayed after I came, who hired him or even what his background was. He'd only show up on day shifts, and never appeared on the work schedule. It was a good thing he didn't see too many patients; he had an interesting habit of giving Demerol intramuscularly to those with head injuries, usually in doses sufficient to make poorly responsive patients, unresponsive.

Shortly after I took my job, at the suggestion of the hospital director, I formed a professional corporation which consisted of me, the chief of dermatology, the chief of surgery, the chief of radiology, and one other. The group wrote a contract with the city to provide health care in the ER. We received a subsidy, and began billing. We never collected much. Because we had a contract with the city, we had to submit a list of employees; their race, sex, and age. The City said there weren't enough minorities among the physicians. No doubt about it. Doctors came to us looking for work based on word of mouth. So I ran an ad in a black medical journal—local to Detroit. I had two responses—both from white physicians; neither of whom had sufficient experience or knowledge to be of any help. One had already retired.

There was never enough room, despite ongoing minor reconstructions. Coming into the ER through the back door (the ambulance dock), the trauma room was on the right, with enough space for about three patients. At the time, it was used only for men. Next, was a small DOA (Dead on Arrival) room, where people who had died on the way to the hospital were taken. Across the hall was a large room in which were crammed as many psychiatric and medical patients as inhumanly possible, waiting for results of tests or to be seen by consultants. Once, I was making rounds, looked into that holding room and saw an ex-governor of Michigan. That is the truth. He got no VIP treatment, and was mixed in with all the other patients. I'm not sure anyone even recognized him.

There were two big rooms, one for men and one for women, meant to hold about twelve patients each. The one for men was used for patients without trauma, including psych patients. The room for women was only for women, including those with trauma and those who were psychiatrically disturbed. In this room, behind curtains that worked on occasion, we did pelvic and rape examinations. The compulsion to separate patients based on their sex, for the sake of privacy was understandable at DGH, where curtains never closed and where it was so crowded that often two patients were in one cubicle. But the compulsion started again at DRH; but we took a strong stand against it. There was little doubt that patients would complain; they didn't.

Between these was another room about six-feet wide that was used for the "overflow." The patients were on gurneys, sometimes squeezed in so tight that the pit boss would have to walk on the gurneys to make rounds, stepping over the patients. The gurneys extended from wall to wall, and from front to back. It was a trick to get in and out of the room.

There were two radiology rooms, but we were decades away from CT scans and MRI's. To do IV studies required a tech or doctor to stay in the room, usually a doctor because techs didn't administer IV's. A cast room, a very small lab and a pediatric section with its own waiting room completed the ER. For the ER, the main hospital lobby, down another corridor, functioned as the waiting area.

Into this chaos I plunged in 1969. I had a relatively free hand at first, as long as I followed basic hospital rules and regulations…and didn't spend a noticeable amount of money…and didn't piss off any of the five unions involved in the ER…and kept the bureaucrats out of it…and, well, you get the picture.

Even today, as I look back, I am not sure why I took this job. I don't regret it; I'm just not sure why I took it. Certainly nothing in my educational background prepared me for what would become an all consuming professional position I had no administrative training, but I was opinionated. And I surely had ideas of what should be done. But I had little idea about how to get them done. Nor did I know of the kinds of interference I would run into. In my own head I had a clear list of objectives and goals to meet.

I didn't and don't know how I got there. I loved medical school and

18

my residency. Actually, I was not crazy about the pre-clinical years, the basic sciences. The clinical years, for me, were fun and invigorating. And the adrenaline rush of my residency was unequaled. The best time of my life was the last two years of medical school and my five years, including internship, of my training would never be rivaled by any other period of my life. Over time, I gained unique stimulation from running codes, especially trauma codes, and being involved in handling the disasters I would face. I liked my patients, in general, and would frequently talk to them about things other than medical problems, and I didn't hesitate to touch them.

My code of ethics, and sense of right and wrong, were an outgrowth of genetics, and environment. I firmly believed that, above all else, to do no harm to those who put their trust and confidence in you. I truly don't remember a time when I didn't want to be a doctor, although my mother wanted me to be a pharmacist so I'd have something to fall back on if I failed in medical school.

The compassion I felt for those injured, ill, or less fortunate, was probably an outgrowth of the deaths of loved ones in my family—my wife and my father—-both of which had a significant impact on me and my life choices.

When I was approached to take this position, I never doubted I could do it, and do it well. I had learned, over time, what had to be changed to make things work. I didn't doubt that these were so obvious, so common sense and such shared goals that everyone would help. God was I wrong.

First, triage systems were set up so patients with minor injuries or illnesses could be seen quickly, and not have to wait, in two rooms up front. A doctor and a nurse moved back and forth between the rooms as quickly as possible, taking care of the chief complaint and referring patients for follow-up. Patients with only dental complaints were sent to dental clinic; those with requests for prescription refills, directly to their clinic, if open. When pediatrics moved to Children's Hospital of Michigan, the space was converted for patients with minor illnesses, an area known as "Screening."

Before an ID system was in place, it wasn't unusual to find dead patients, unknown to the nursing and medical staff, on gurneys. Or have the wrong patient transferred out; or the wrong body, taken to the morgue; or the wrong patient, given a blood transfusion.

The task of getting and making sure all patients had ID bracelets was much more arduous than it should have been. Gaining consensus for the bracelet color was a major challenge, as was getting money to buy them — and getting the clerks to apply them. The clerical staff was really resistant to applying the wrist tags. They looked at it as an added job. All they had to do was apply the tag and write the patient's name and number on it. I regret to say that theirs was a typical city employee response to a new task; one they didn't regularly have to do.

Screens were put up on the windows, which freed us from flying, but not crawling, vermin. The crawling vermin were always with us; sometimes within a day or two of the exterminator.

Roaches in back we need an exterminator
Entry: 8/14/78
Hygiene problem worse today ice machine loaded with roaches.
Entry: 8/15/78
Floater: JMN
Rat killed (DIE) in meditation room.
Entry: 10/07/80
Floater: BFB
Mice in OCU
Entry: 10/6/81
Floater: Krome

Even at DRH rats were a problem. The health department was called by unknown individuals when rats were found wandering on the ambulance dock.

We began hiring our own attending physicians; some full time. All moonlighters had their quality of care reviewed and, since they were one of the rare groups without a union contract, we could fire them with ease, notifying their residency director.

An occasional full timer was trouble. One guy was often late or missed shifts. I became convinced; although I couldn't prove it, that he was a drinking man. Eventually, I didn't renew his contract and he went to the west coast. But I did speak to the guy who hired him.

It wasn't rare for moonlighters to just blow off a shift entirely and not show up. No more. Those who didn't show up just once were told not to bother showing up again. Late comers had their pay docked.

The attendings wore long white coats, generally over green scrubs. Residents wore the same outfit, while medical students wore short white costs over their greens, or civilian clothes under the coats. Although we tried to encourage everyone to dress nicely, and wear civilian clothes under their white coats, it was impossible. Sooner or later in every shift they either were vomited on, urinated on or soaked in blood. So everyone wore clothes that could be changed easily during the shift and shoes they didn't care about.

Emergency-specific educational programs were begun on a regular basis for residents, students, nurses and attendings.

The ER became a closed nursing unit, which meant that we had our own nursing supervisor and our own specialized criteria for nurses. Our nurses could no longer be pulled to work on the wards when they were short handed; but we couldn't get help from them either.

There were morning staff meetings before 1974, as early as 1969, but recorded history didn't begin until 1974. Initially, attendance included the senior physician (floater), the on-coming shift nursing supervisor, or head nurse, the off-going shift nursing supervisor, and the chief of the registration personnel. Representatives of other departments came as the need for the exchange of information to resolve problems expanded. Rape counseling, social services, psychiatry, pharmacy, and security, eventually began coming. In the infrastructure of the ER, and the hospital, this meeting assumed an extremely important position. On rare occasions senior hospital administrative staff showed up, especially the vice-president to whom I reported.

As time went on, I was unavoidably and increasingly entangled with the hospital bureaucracy. More rewardingly, I became a strong advocate for improved emergency care and heavily involved in the expanding role of emergency medicine on a state, regional and national level.

I remained dedicated to bettering conditions and care for our own ER patients. It was, moreover, my primary job. To make sure I was up-to-date on the daily goings on, morning staff meetings to review the previous day's concerns and prepare for the day's events were held; a problem solving meeting.

The meetings were run by the senior emergency physician coming on that morning. Among this lucky doctor's other responsibilities was recording the various and sundry information about his or her day— which included twelve hours on site and twelve hours on call from home—in a running logbook.

This doc had no specific room assignment, but helped wherever needed, the position became known as the "floater" and the logbook became the "floater's log." The floater had to also help with administrative and nursing problems. He was the expediter calling consultants and helping get patients to their hospital beds. Over time the floaters not only recorded problems that required resolution, but also, incidents and events of general interest.

It was to fifteen years' worth of floater's logs that I turned to write this book. No one had written in it with the intention of creating a literary gem, or even leaving a lasting impression. But that's just what they did.

I can still feel the same frustration and anger I felt when originally reading each note: frustration with a system that treated poor people poorly and with those who lacked the vision or courage to change, and frustration over my own inability to get others to see what was really going on. I can feel it even now, remembering the times when I and other doctors were moved to tears over what was, and was not, happening. One of my colleagues aptly said, "Receiving was the best second class hospital in the country."

And yet, with the help of those who did care, doctors, nurses, pharmacists, social workers, chaplains, laboratory personnel, housekeepers and others — people to whom I owe my career and this book — a difference was made. With little, they did much.

There were two things which occurred when I was an intern which help demonstrate the nature and personality of the hospital. The first occurred shortly after I started on my first rotation through the emergency room. I was really naïve even though in my head I was sophisticated. One evening when I was working before there was triage, the police wheeled in a patient in a dress and long hair. They were rolling towards the male trauma room when I stopped them. "Guys, she belongs in room twelve (the female room)."

The officers broke out in a big smile. "No we aren't. She is a he." My first contact with a transvestite. Not my last.

I was working in room twelve when a woman was brought in after a seizure, frothing at the mouth, with blood running out. We all assumed she had bitten her tongue. We pried her mouth open and removed a "lump" of tissue, which turned out to be the end of a man's penis. I put it in a sterile saline wrap, while others treated her for her seizure. I ran up the hall to the male trauma room, where doctors were examining a man's blood soaked crotch, missing a piece of his penis. "I think you guys need this," and handed them the missing part.

It seems that the woman was performing fellatio on the man when she sustained her seizure. Both survived their sexual encounter.

Again, I was in room twelve, I saw and examined a young lady with a big protuberant tummy. She had no menses in the past six months. She described the pain as intermittent and cramping. She had had unprotected intercourse (no one used condoms in those days). Pregnancy test meant that a frog had to die or a rabbit get pregnant. No fast pregnancy tests. I did a rectal examine (pelvic examination had either to be sterile or require a setup for impending pregnancy). I felt the cervix which was elongated and open about four centimeters. I in my wisdom was convinced that she was in labor. So I called the gyn resident. He didn't think she was, but admitted her. When I got my follow up information, about a week later, I was told she wasn't pregnant. She had a pancreatic cyst, very large; had it drained and did well.

The confidence I had when I left medical school was waning.

Chapter II
The Beginning

In the beginning was the word, and the word was "floater."

This is the first effective date of the new enlarged policy for the physician assigned to the position of floater.

Entry: May 5, 1974

Floater: JNM

Floater

An emergency physician will be assigned daily to the floater position.

Upon reporting for duty, he will notify the nursing supervisor and the administrative duty officer.

At anytime that he leaves the Emergency Department, he will notify the operator of his location (we didn't have pagers or beepers at that time).

The floater will make rounds periodically throughout the entire Department, but at least hourly in the O.C.U. (Observation Care Unit-a specifically constructed unit of eighteen beds designed to hold patients while they waited for a bed in the hospital, got prolonged emergency treatment to prevent their hospitalization, or psychiatrically disturbed patients, waiting or receiving continual therapy).

He will insure that each treatment area is adequately staffed. Should additional nursing staff be required, he will notify the nursing supervisor. Should additional medical staff be required, he will provide help himself.

He will provide medical support whenever any treatment area falls behind.

He will know the location of all members of the medical staff at all times, making sure that coffee and lunch breaks are not prolonged.

He will insure that all physicians report for work on time and stay their entire shift.

Monday through Friday, he will attend at 6:00 am; he will attend the morning staff meeting held in the ED conference room.

He will insure that all patients are seen promptly by consultants.

Nursing supervisors, administrative duty officers and consulting staff are to take their problems to the floater.

Upon completion of his shift, he will make a note in the Floater's Log which will be the kept in ADO. Office (Administrative Duty Officer). The note should include, but not be limited to, the following information:

Unusual and/or problem cases (patient's name, unit number, and problem.

Names of physicians who were late and/or those that didn't show.

Non-medical staffing problems.

Unusual delays in x-ray and /or lab.

Any unusual incidents.

The floater's name.

EFFECTIVE DATE: 5/74

MM referred from Detox (Alcohol Detoxification Center) *for suicide attempt. Walked out. Discussed at morning report.*
Entry: 5/16/74
Floater: JNB

Psychiatrically disturbed, or intoxicated, patients frequently walked out of the ER. We notified police and family to be on the look out, and, if indicated, the facility which had sent the patient. Because of the high incidence of elopements, the policy of having patients held only under direct nursing staff observation was instituted. Now it seems that such a policy shouldn't even have been a topic of discussion. Nursing shortages meant this often didn't happen. Nurses didn't like baby sitting and the techs would often wander off, leaving patients alone.

Another fire in room one yesterday. More often than not room one is without staff, despite there being a room assignment. It's getting common to find pts. (Patients) *on the floor, or half out of their stretchers* (gurneys) *& no nurse or attendant in room.*
Entry: 2/19/75
Floater: JET

DGH had one of the few psychiatric crisis centers in the city, so we got virtually every patient who tried, or threatened to try, to commit suicide. A lot of people. Patients requiring hospitalization were admitted or transferred to a state psychiatric facility. In the late '80s, the state entered a cost saving mode, closing the state psychiatric facilities or limiting their admissions.

Because of what I interpreted as the best interests of the patients, both those mentally challenged (regardless of the cause), and those not so challenged, whenever we received a patient who could not care for themselves, they were restrained with leather restraint straps; either one hand and one leg or all four extremities; never across the abdomen or chest. This was not humane but it certainly prevented patients from wandering around, stealing from other patients, disrupting staff, or otherwise having or causing problems.

Michigan's treatment of its psychiatric citizens was appalling. And we were certainly part of the problem; we were the intake point of so many of these unfortunate people. Although changes did occur over time, it wasn't until the '90's that things improved. These patients made up ten percent of our volume but ninety perecent of our problems. Virtually every week we made the papers about our psych patients, and their problems.

Periodically, a new physician would become especially incensed by our restraint policy. In fact they would refuse to place these patients in restraints. On one such occasion, the nursing boss told me that a released patient, suicidal, had escaped. The physician never did it again!

At a news conference, when we were talking about the volume of psych patients and our problems with the load, a reporter asked me what made the volume go so high. I facetiously said that it may be because of the full moon. Needless to say, they ran that quote, and I received calls from astrologists who wanted to caste my horoscope.

There were two health reporters in Detroit I respected enormously, each worked for one of the daily newspapers in Detroit, in the days when we actually had two different newspapers; each approached health care problems from a different perspective. The lady worked for the Detroit Free Press was more exposure oriented, tending to take stories out to their most sensational endpoint. The other reporter, who worked for the Detroit News, was more scholarly, slower in the development of his stories, and more prone to do in depth stories. They were both extremely competent and most of us in health care had a great deal of respect for each of them.

The News reporter came to see me, without an appointment. Neither reporter required one; my secretary was smart enough to know who they were and what they could mean to us. SC, the reporter, said he had a great story idea and needed my help. He wanted to do an in depth piece about psychiatric care, and wanted to be committed to NSH, a state psychiatric facility. SC wanted to start like all patients in our crisis center.

My job was to give him a list of symptoms he was to have, and to insure that the staff, many of whom knew him, would not blow the whistle. How he would get discharged was his problem. So one day, unannounced, he showed up brought in by police. SC spent two days strapped to a gurney before he was sent to NSH (Northville State

Hospital) by ambulance. His story was great. It certainly made an impact. In fact, we would sometimes use these two reporters to leak stories that could help us. I never lied to them and always answered their questions truthfully.

We kept gallon jugs of pHisohex, Maalox, and aspirins. There were a lot of alcoholics with gastric disturbances treated with Maalox, a milky white solution looking like pHisohex. Both were kept in the same cabinet; right next to each other, not smart. One drunk, not restrained, got off his gurney, went to the cabinet and helped himself to a large paper cup filled with pHisohex, thinking it was Maalox, before he was caught. I don't know how, but he didn't get sick. I guess the old saying, "God takes care of fools and drunks," is true.

We kept three different colors of aspirins-yellow, green and blue. No other over the counter analgesics. And patients generally knew, and would swear they got relief from a specific colored aspirin, and would only take that color. "Give me the green aspirins, Doc."

EM – overweight 550-600 pounds. Difficult placement. Finally found place in Wayne County Extended Care facility. Surgery not interested in doing anything surgical treatment of obesity.
   Entry: 5/16/74
   Floater: JM

EM was neither the first nor the last patient seen with medical problems and morbid obesity. She was bedridden for almost six years. When the ambulance arrived, it took six to eight attendants to transfer her to a gurney. She was moved to a treatment area (room twelve). A work-up was begun and she waited for x-ray. We decided to x-ray her on the gurney, but while waiting, she fell off. The staff stood back, looking at each other waiting for someone to make a decision.

There was silence in the room. SB, a senior medical attendant finally said, "I'll take care of it, Dr. Krome." He left, returning five to ten minutes later, riding a high low, with a morgue gurney on the front. He and several other attendants rolled EM on to the morgue gurney, and SB raised her, on the high low and rolled her onto the two gurneys strapped together. She never once complained.

When her workup was complete, she was treated for heart failure. There was still the problem of where she could go for continuing care. Her family couldn't, or wouldn't, care for her at home. They had already spent six years watching her lie in bed and gain weight. We finally found an extended care facility to take her. I never saw her again. But I am sure that she didn't have a long, happy life.

This was the time before surgical intervention for morbid obesity was popular. The surgical consultants didn't want to take any chances and operate on her. I didn't blame them.

Problems today
Patient JB BS (blood sugar=10) we called lab and were told it was on wrong patient. BS was really 93.
Entry: 5/22/74
Floater: JET

A blood sugar of ten is a critical level, and associated with significant complications, including death. JB was alert, clear and coherent, and without seizures. This compelled the doctor to check with the lab regarding the results. No one from the lab had called to alert the physician of this critical level. It turned out to be some other patient's results.

Lab errors weren't terribly unusual, not common just not unusual. I was taught by a mentor one of the great truths I would live by in medicine. "If the lab results don't match what you clinically see or hear, redo the lab." In years to come, I would teach this to my students and residents.

Patient SH arrived 5/22/74 on citation sent to psych who felt that patient had OBS (Organic Brain Syndrome). History not compatible.
Entry: 5/24/74
Floater: JET

SH was reevaluated in the medical treatment area; including having a LP (spinal tap). She had an elevated protein and elevated white blood cells. Tests for tuberculosis, and cultures were obtained. The physician felt the patient might have encephalitis, and consultation was requested from both neurology and internal medicine. By the morning of the twenty-fourth, no one had come to see the patient, so the patient was transferred to Hutzel Hospital, one of our sister hospitals, where she was admitted.

Obtaining consultations was a continuing problem. There were certain specialties that gave the impression ER patients were low on their priority list. In the 2000's it started to improve. There were long delays in obtaining a consultation, except from the emergency surgery services, which had someone stationed in the ER, most of the time. The process of getting a decision from a consultant was convoluted and time consuming.

It went something like this: first response by a junior resident or senior student, who evaluates patient and orders additional laboratory tests and x-rays. Delay in getting results. First responder returns to see test results, then calls next resident up the line, who comes to see patient and checks results, adding additional tests. He comes back to recheck results. Then, calls the next resident up the line; they usually make a decision on the phone. On some services, the attending physician is also contacted. If it was surgery, the attending physician, who slept in the hospital, came to see the patient. If patient was admitted, a bed had to be found. Finally, there were some wards, with a lack of adequately trained nursing staff on midnights, to which the residents were reluctant to admit truly sick or injured patients. I supported this decision. God, I don't know how we did it.

I was working trauma when a patient with massive hemoptysis (coughing up blood), probably from active tuberculosis, arrived. I couldn't stop the bleeding and needed help from someone more knowledgeable. I paged the cardio-thoracic fellow, who told me that their consults were first seen by the surgery resident working trauma. I turned and saw it was one of our own junior emergency medicine residents. This wasn't satisfactory to me. Either he came or I would call his staff. He came. The patient was taken to the OR and survived.

I once studied the time it took to make a final decision, from patient's arrival to the consultant's final decision. The combination of psychiatric and internal medicine consultations was the worst. These two together would fairly routinely bring the time up to in excess of twenty-four hours. Of course, just psych consult would eat up the most time. All the while, the patient laid on a gurney with a two-inch foam mattress, eating one meal a day——consisting of a "Kromeburger,"—- with infrequent trips to the restrooms, and little or no water. We were really inhumane. We did good medical work; but humane patient service was less than desired.

In an attempt to speed up the process of admission, and decrease the waiting time in the ER, the medical executive committee (the ruling medical body) passed a rule that patients could only stay a maximum of twenty-four hours in the ER from arrival until either admission or discharge. This wasn't exactly what I wanted, but it was a suitable compromise. Time started when the patient entered the ER. When the twenty-four hours ended the patient had to be admitted or discharged. Working on the assumption that the consultant knew more than me about patient's medical problems, and admission was safer than discharge, patients were all admitted to the last service responsible for him. Our admissions clerks had to notify the admitting service. Even though not every service was happy about this, it certainly expedited movement of ER patients.

Patient EM......deaf Spanish lady...'
Entry in log 5/23/74
Floater: JET

EM, a "little old lady, deaf Spanish-speaking lady," who spoke no English, was picked up by the police and brought to us. The police and later, EMS brought all lost persons to us. In the early 1960s, we could arrange to check missing persons and run the patient's fingerprints through the armed service files and the FBI files, leading us to find the patient's name and address. In the late '60s, fingerprint files became inaccessible. So our social worker had to spend a good deal of time locating the point of origin of the patient.

This patient had been picked up two doors from her home. Because she was old, couldn't communicate, and used a foreign language, which the police assumed was gibberish she was brought in as a lost person. It took until 5:23 a.m. the next day to figure it out. The other languages we had trouble with were Polish and Slavic. To this list, today you can add Arabic. Even though we have interpreters, their availability and our demand did not always match.

We had two groups of elderly patients. The first are dropped off by friends or family at the ambulance door and taken to the Triage station. Their families want us to find a place for them to live, and don't want to be involved themselves. These were the geriatric dumplings. Sometimes the police or EMS will do the dumping. It might take us hours to complete the workup and arrange for placement.

The second were geriatric foundlings, unidentified and "lost" on the streets, frequently homeless, uninsured and with no one to turn to for help. It seemed to me then and now, that we were the only hospital in the country that served as a tracer of lost persons.

One time, in the '80s, a room and board facility was closed down and the five elderly persons who lived there, now without a place to live, were brought to our ED (Emergency Department), as a group. The accompanying worker told us what happened and that we had to find a place for them to live. It made all the Detroit papers, and eventually the social work staff at DRH resolved the issue.

Incident with Mr. M...already reported
Entry: 5/23/74
Floater: JET

Not self defense. In Mr. M's mind, this required retaliation.

He filed a union grievance. I really didn't want to fire him or suspend him. Mr. M was one of our medical attendants. I really liked him. He was generally jovial and gregarious, and usually followed the rules, although he had trouble taking orders from the registered nurses responsible for supervising him. I really don't think he liked taking orders from women and all of our RN's were women. In fact, authority figures gave him heart burn and raised his adrenaline levels. Anger management was not Mr. M's strong suit.

On this day, or the day before, he was suspended for striking a patient. Not that we were against self defense, but this one was restrained all four (arms and legs) to a gurney. He spit on Mr. M, who retaliated by striking the patient. But I had no choice. I discussed the problem with the ER nursing director, and we both agreed that if he accepted transfer to another department, with low patient contact, we would be alright, and the hospital would still have a reasonable employee.

Before the grievance meeting, the union steward approached me, or I her, and we talked. I told her about our proposal to transfer Mr. M. Since this was a first time occurrence, ten days and firing was harsh, but she might be open to transfer him, depending on what happened in the meeting. Mr. M lost his temper, and began shouting and yelling. We adjourned, and the union steward agreed with the transfer. He went to the OR, and as I understand he functioned very well. Often, he would come down to talk. I never detected any animosity.

Chapter III

3:50 pm
1. Patient brought to court (located across the street from Receiving)
2. Patient passed out in court. Brought to DGH
3. Seen in room 7 and referred to Psych
4. Patient ran out of room 7 and out of DGH
5. Patient intercepted by me on corner St. Antoine and Clinton
6. Patient returned to DGH & turned over to psych and room 15 staff
7. Patient ran out of psych room and out of room 15 and out of DGH
8. ADO (Administrative Duty Officer) notified to call police regarding patient escape
Entry: 6/18/74
Floater: MJN

MJN was a meticulous floater. He was one of the first full-timers I hired. His notes were very much like entries made by a military officer, which he was. Over time, he began having difficulty staying

34

up with changes in medicine, especially the changes in emergency medicine practice. MJN was mostly hindered by his conservatism. He really liked the status quo, and worked hard to keep it. Of Greek-American extraction, his family had land in Greece which he periodically visited; he would return with olive oil and wine as gifts. Once, there was a coup attempt in Greece, according to N., Greece wasn't really ready for democracy!

As time went on, MJN became more unresponsive when paged. We didn't have beepers, but all floaters were told they had to keep the ER and the hospital operators aware of how to be reached when not in the hospital. Added to his problems were his long lunches and time away when actually on duty. Eventually, I had no choice but to terminate his employment, despite the fact that he had become a shareholder. The other senior emergency physicians asked me over and over again to do this. I resisted because he had been there from the beginning, when times were really tough, and I felt some loyalty to him. I even tried to talk him into retiring. Nothing worked so I let him go. He sued me and the corporation for wrongful discharge. We settled out of court.

DOA GSW to heart (Dead on Arrival) age 11
Entry; 6/25/74
Floater: JNM

JNM was saddled with the responsibility of telling the family of the death of this child. Eleven. Shot on the streets of Detroit, a random shooting from a car driven by teenagers. In the '60s, an Army guy, just back from 'Nam, was shot on the streets of Detroit. Killed. Survived 'Nam, just came home, walking to visit family, in his uniform, and was killed. Survived a year in 'Nam, but not a day in Detroit. Parents shouldn't survive their kids. It is just too unconscionable; too much grief. Children killing children.

DOA's were patients who arrived dead and on whom we didn't/couldn't work. Resuscitation was out of the question. They arrived without a heart beat, no breathing, pupils fixed and dilated. Mostly they

35

were trauma deaths; but some had medical problems, chronic ones, those whose time had run out. If they were warm and had even a slight pulse, we would try. If they were kids, no matter what, the staff would still try.

At times our efforts took a long time. Patients who suffered from hypothermia (cold exposure producing a decrease in body temperature) and had a cardiac arrest required a prolonged resuscitation with increasingly complicated methods to warm them. Those who had cancer and were terminal you let go. You had to know and learn when enough was enough. Sometimes even the most experienced of us couldn't let go. Maybe the patient reminded us of a family member or friend who had died, and we didn't want to watch it again. Of course, there were the very old. They were ready. You could see it in their eyes; see it in their body language. You knew they were ready to die. They had made peace and were prepared.

Today, patients and or their families are more involved in the decision making process. Power of attorney, and "do not resuscitate" papers are available more often. But you had to be suspicious when a family member, or an alleged family member, told you that the patient didn't want to be resuscitated, or have heroic efforts done. I have almost been caught when it turned out that the next of kin couldn't prove it, or there was no written expression of the patient's wishes. Cynically, you had to follow the money!

When I was a senior medical student, on neurosurgery I had my first professional encounter with death. We had a patient, a man, with a family, including kids, how many I can't remember. He had just come down from the operating room and was in the NICU (Neurosurgical Intensive Care Unit). The tumor he had couldn't be resected, and his skull couldn't be closed because there was too much brain swelling.

The neurosurgery residents had a departmental party. I was left in charge, so to speak. I was to call the on-call resident right after I pronounced the patient or if I had any problems. The patient was going to die sometime that night. The family had been informed and was waiting. There were to be no heroic efforts.

I was scared and insecure. This was the first time I had the responsibility of pronouncing a real patient; someone I had responsibility for, even though very limited. I sat at the nurses' station waiting for the Angel of Death to make his rounds. Periodically, I would go to the bedside and check the patient. Finally, there was no pulse, no respirations and no pupil reflexes. The cardiac monitor went off; the piercing sound. The family never took their eyes off me.

I immediately called a colleague of mine who was also on-call. I heard stories of patients being pronounced, and suddenly sitting up either in the morgue or en route. This sure as hell wasn't going to happen to me. My colleague arrived, listened to the patient's heart, and nodded. I told the family. They thanked both of us. I am not sure if they ever knew how afraid or insecure I was.

. One night, during my internship, I, had to pronounce a patient I was truly responsible for. I still see and hear him after all these years. I was called because the patient was having trouble breathing. He was a heavy set white man, with a pot belly. He was sitting up in bed, first bed in the first ward on unit 4-1. The ward was a twenty-two bed unit with curtains for privacy.

It was night, I am not sure exactly when, but it seems, as I look back, that most of these things happened after the sun went down. The patient was in obvious respiratory distress; no chest pain. His lungs sounded like congestive failure. His color was still good. This was in late 1961 or early 1962.

There were a lot of limitations in our medicine chest. There were no statins; no daily aspirin; no lasix; no cardiac enzymes; and no beta blockers. By today's standards, we were a third world nation. We got a portable chest x-ray and an EKG. No myocardial infarction on EKG. Pulmonary effusion on chest x-ray.

He was given morphine sulfate, aminophylline, and was started on rotating tourniquets. I called the resident for help. Got none. I was doing what was standard for the time. He was going downhill; in the medical vernacular' he was circling the drain.

He looked me straight in the eye:

Am I going to die?

I was caught twixt the devil and a hard place. I didn't want to lie to him; but I didn't want to tell him the truth either. It was time I learned the proverbial two steps:

Not if I can help it

You can't

Shortly, it was over. He died. I called out the time for the nurse and went to the desk to sit and stew and rethink everything. I sat in my sweat, my scrubs drenched. I made the calls I had to make, the next of kin and the medical examiner. The family wouldn't sign for an autopsy. Something I didn't like to ask for anyhow. The medical examiner released the body and I signed the death certificate.

I really thought when I entered medical school; I'd be able to make a difference. I never pictured myself pronouncing people dead. They hadn't taught much about death; just when life was over. None of the moral or ethical dilemmas we faced when death came. I was learning how difficult it was to do battle with the Angel of Death. Sometimes he won; sometimes you won. But it was always associated with a load of adrenaline and sometimes prayer.

I am not an especially religious man. I believe in God, but not organized religion. But in the resuscitation room, when we are all working on a patient and trying to sustain or save a life, when it is quiet and everyone is thinking of the next step after a long series of steps, when everything has failed, I can hear him, the flapping of his wings. The angel of death has come to collect. I look up at the head of the bed, where the respirator is and can see, really see, him. I know it sounds superstitious and borderline psychotic, but I do. I know it is over. I believe.

My father died, as I said elsewhere, when I was eighteen. Sometime later, I am not sure when I started to see him. I always talked to him, but never saw him until then. It started when I would look into the mirror and see his face where mine was. Then, overtime I would see him standing there, especially at night when I was outside smoking. Things would go well for me and I knew he was my guardian angel. About four years ago, after I became semi-retired, I was standing outside in the early morning hours and I felt a tug on my shirt sleeve. I turned and saw my father, smiling, smoking a cigar, and waving goodbye. I have never seen him again. I don't know if it was as a result of the therapy I was in, or a natural progression. I still talk to him.

I know I am a depressive, but I really have trouble dealing with death. I don't like it and I can't even bring myself to go to funerals.

There were times when the battle seemed so senseless; like the eleven-year-old shot on the street; like the vet who just returned from 'Nam shot walking to his mother's house the day after he returned; like the family of five wiped out by a drunk driver who came in for us to work on; and like the druggies who overdosed. It could be frustrating and difficult to maintain a professional demeanor. Everyone was approached as though they were the president of the United States, but there were some the nurses couldn't even talk to.

There were those who came in ready to die. Like the sixty-year-old man, trapped in an apartment fire, who suffered a one hundred percent body burn, who requested he not be resuscitated. Nowadays, they would have "no code" papers. (Now, called "Do not resuscitate" orders). Some even wait at home until the last minute. Families don't like to watch their loved ones fade away peacefully even when it is expected. I'm not sure, even today, that families know what to do, so they call 911. It appears as though they must have their family members brought to the temple—to the hospital- - to make their final stop on earth, before they could die.

When we see them, when we look into their eyes, we see peace and preparation to meet their Maker. They are ready to go, and we shouldn't get in the way.

Facing death is never easy. Whether it is someone you care for, or someone for whom you are caring, or your own. Many people think physicians are insensitive, withdrawn, indifferent, and cold when it comes to dealing with death. There are times when physicians do put up strong defensive measures; but you never really get used to it.

I finished medical school in 1961. There were no courses or lectures about death. The goal of medical school was to teach us to diagnose and treat diseases and injuries; to save lives, or prolong life.

I never learned anything about interpersonal relations surrounding this area. I had learned things when I had to deal with death in my own family, my father and my first wife. Surprisingly, I found talking to my rabbi helpful in trying to understand my father's death.

When he died, our rabbi came to talk to my brother and me; my brother was sixteen, I was eighteen. I remember it like it was yesterday. We had just said our morning and mourning prayers. We sat in straight back chairs. My mother and sister were in the other room.

The secret to getting into heaven, according to him, was the living. The souls of those who died were in limbo, awaiting the decision regarding their fate. The single biggest factor, that influenced God the most, was whether someone loved them and remembered them after they died. And the measure of that was saying the mourning prayer each day for the year. There was no way to test this theory. We weren't going to take any chances. So we said the prayers each and every day for a year; then on each anniversary of his death. Our remembrance of him was his key to heaven. I am sure this little homily was told by our rabbi to all his young congregants who lost family. I loved it and over time modified it and used it when talking to family.

No health care provider likes facing death, especially his own. This may be one psychological factor influencing our choice of specialties. Surely, there are specialties that limit our contact with death, or sick people. Perhaps, we enter medical school to not deal with death. We think we are protected from our own death because of our chosen profession. Somehow, being a doctor protects us from death or sickness.

As I went through residency, I watched others facing this daunting task. Over time I adopted some of what they said and did. Another factor influencing me was a monologue by a famous comedian. He spoke about the words doctors used to break the bad news. I used to say the same things.

Doctor: We lost your husband

Family: Where did you put him? That's horrible.

Doctor: Your husband didn't make it.

Family: I saw him put on the ambulance. Did they have an accident? Did they go to the wrong hospital?

Doctor: Your husband expired

Like a credit card; like a library card?

These are the usual euphemisms to keep from using the words: "death" or "dead"; protecting us. Hoping it works.

All of this helps us in grieving; in not feeling guilty about our potential inadequacy in not saving the patient. Many residents have come to me after a death asking if there was anything they could have done differently. One good reason for mortality and morbidity conferences is it helps us face our own responsibility in case management. We all have to grieve. We all have to recognize our responsibility to and for the patient.

Chapter IV
Transfer from St. Joe's

Received transfer from St. Joe's at 8:00AM...
Received from St. Joe's at 8:00 AM. Stab 3rd. ICS (intercostals space) with 50% pneumo (pneumothorax=air in the chest which didn't belong there) *identified by them prior to transfer. Patient arrived without O2, IV, or chest tube.*
Entry: 9/15/74
Floater: W.

Three years later, W. had another bad transfer.

AS 926026 elderly white male was transferred from Southwest...with a dx of "R/O ruptured aortic aneurysm." Transfer was made without acceptance after our surgical resident told SWG this diagnosis made it presumptive pt. was unstable for to transfer. Pt. arrived in full cardiac arrest (v fib) and was resuscitated. Admitted to E. Surg
Entry: 3/9/77
Floater: W.

JF—Pt. drove himself from D........ Hosp. with a transfer slip, IV, and fx orbit.

Entry: 3/21/77
Floater: BFB
St. J...called this am to transfer pt. RH. ADO refused. St. J...sent pt. anyway. DGH sent pt. back. Called administrator (Mrs. C.) to tell her of situation. She assured me it wouldn't happen again.
Entry: 5/1/76
Floater: BFB

Although we didn't often send patients back, unannounced transfers were reaching enormous proportions. So we started. Once I denied a transfer and a doc proceeded to lambaste me. He wanted to transfer an uninsured patient. He told me I had no choice, that the city charter obligated us to take all patients in transfer. I told him he had us confused with Wayne County General Hospital and hung up on him. I didn't need someone to teach me my responsibility to the community.

1 transfer from Metro Hospital in Windsor Res in N/S (neurosurgery) called & accepted
Entry: 3/20/81
Floater: JMN

Windsor, Ontario, located about three to four miles from DRH had a working relationship with us. Windsor only had two neurosurgeons, and when they both were out of town, we accepted their patients. This was an interesting arrangement. There was nothing in writing since such a written agreement could be construed as an international treaty, which would require congressional approval.

Transfers to us were not unusual, and, not often preceded by a telephone call; some patients required a rapid response. He was started on oxygen, two IV's were started, a portable chest x-ray obtained (which confirmed the presence of the pneumothorax), a chest tube inserted and the patient admitted. Sometimes patients arrived without a transfer note; sometimes, they did, recounting what had been done at the sending hospital. This was in the seventies, by the eighties, this had changed. In 1977, transfers of patients from one major hospital were so often unstable that we kept a separate record of their transfers. Calls were made; transfers accepted or rejected; transfer notes sent.

Prior to Roe v. Wade, we received numerous unannounced female patients in sepsis, or shock, from a septic abortion. When I started my training, we had sixty gynecology beds; almost all filled with women who had septic abortions—illegal abortions. And illegal abortions were not uncommon. Sometimes the abortion was self-induced with a hanger, a pencil, or potassium permanganate solution as a douche. There was a secret list of physicians who might accept pregnant patients for abortions. By the time they were septic, we couldn't refer them. All patients who had an incomplete abortion or a septic abortion required a D & C; usually under IV sedation and local anesthesia. One night I, an intern, and my gyn resident did five in a row; sometimes I did it, sometimes he did it. First he put in the local anesthetic, and I would do the D & C. I would put in the anesthetic and he would do the procedure.

Although we felt a great sense of pride in being the hospital who "took all comers" regardless of ability to pay, we felt an overwhelming pressure at being the conscience of the community and much abused by the City, its citizens, and other hospitals. When patients had no insurance or money, they flocked to us; when they did they flew to other hospitals, as though we didn't accept insurance or money!

Covering for President Gerald Ford today.
Room 2 set up (shock trauma room)
Anesthesiology set to cover.
EMS coordinated.
Entry: 10/10/74
Floater: M.

DRH was the primary response hospital whenever a visiting dignitary came to Detroit. Wayne County General hospital served in this capacity from the landing at Detroit Metropolitan Airport until the city limits were reached by the motorcade. Then we took responsibility. Even now (2004) we function in this capacity. There is no more Wayne County General.

The process was very involved. Medical information was not given to us because it was considered classified; but we managed to get some answers. Generally, the process began with an inspection by the Secret Service, who checked out the hospital and made sure we would have a surgical, neurosurgical, and orthopedic attending on scene. The location of the blood bank, OR, and ICU's were noted, while they made plans to insure security of all locations. A white security phone with a ring down to the White House switchboard was placed at the nurses' station. Evidently we forgot to tell one of ward clerks what the phone was for, and how it should be answered. Since the president hadn't arrived yet, the agent assigned to the phone wasn't there when it rang. The ward clerk picked it up on its first ring.

White House Switchboard.
Clerk: Who?
Whitehouse Switchboard.
Clerk: Who the hell is this?
White House Switchboard
Clerk: Don't play me. I got work to do.
White House Switchboard
Clerk: I ain't got time to fuck with you, asshole.

Down went the phone. Immediately an agent appeared, but no one got in trouble.

An EMS rig followed the motorcade with a doctor, and our Police Huey (helicopter) flew over it into the City. The helicopter had police officers, a secret service agent, a doctor and a nurse on board. The agent had no sense of humor and never took his eyes off the window, always watching.

There was a security meeting before each visit; attended by secret service, police, fire, FBI, and the Chief of EMS. The chief of EMS invited me to come. Curious as hell, I went. I was stunned by the lack of security at the security meeting. Remember this was in the seventies. I hope things are much tighter now. In any case, no one checked my ID. I sat next to the chief, while the secret service reviewed ID lapel pins for all security, the place in the motorcade of the president's car, the location of snipers placed by them, and the motorcade route. Thank God I wasn't running black ops——merely a curious doc.

A lot of our responsibilities for VIP'S came to ahead when the Republican National Convention was held in Detroit in the summer of 1980. Many, many VIP'S came in for the convention. Some came with their own medical staff; some with secret service coverage. Our medical information was limited at best. The hospital was setup as I said before, and was ready everyday, twenty-four hours a day, for the duration of the convention. Paramedics and nurses, again volunteers, patrolled the convention floor and the seating areas. A first aid station was set up in the convention arena. In addition, a fire rescue vehicle, set up as a mobile emergency room, was parked next to the convention site. I even got to drive it from the hospital to the convention site at twenty-five miles an hour. I was impressed! With all this medical support, we had virtually nothing more medically necessary than Tylenol.

Every time there was a convention of some sort we were put on alert, as was EMS. We met with the organizers of the convention, I in my dual capacity as medical director of EMS and chief of emergency medicine. Frequently we asked for volunteers to staff the convention center. When there was a Boy Scout jamboree on Belle Isle, we asked for volunteers to staff it and stay on the island.

Chapter V
First Day of LPN Strike

*First day of strike by LPN's (*licensed practical nurses*) &*
supporters
Entry 11/18/74
Floater: M.

The rumor mill had been working that the LPN's were going to
walk out; I am not sure it was ever an official strike. In addition to the
LPN's, the RN's, medical attendants, supervisory nurses, registration
personnel were all unionized. All had labor contracts with the City,
which were periodically renegotiated. Most of the time, when they
went out it was for money. Sometimes they wanted additional
education or health benefits. When the LPN's went out they protested
right outside the hospital and picketed on the sidewalks. All city
operated clinics were affected.

We still saw patients in the ED; RN's and supervisory personnel
had to pitch in and help. The mayor of the city made them an offer, and
then allegedly said that if they weren't back in three days he would fire
them all. I don't know if he actually said it or not. I do know they were
back in three days.

Fantastic blizzard
Entry: 12/1/74
Floater: T.

This was the great blizzard of 1974. I can't remember how much snow we got, but I know it was a helluva a lot. All non essential people were sent home. Offices were closed; city buildings closed; streets, roadways, expressways were all closed and impassable. Nurses, attendants, and doctors couldn't get in to work.

"I wished I could have spent the evening building snowpersons (snowman is a sexist term)." T.

DIE (died in emergency) cardiac arrest...
Entry: 12/14/74
Floater: B.

Most of what we did, we did well, very well. However, we weren't perfect. Approximately ninety-five percent of those who arrived alive left alive. Not all survived their hospitalizations. Sometimes we just didn't do things right. Or sometimes the gods were against us and the patient.

This evening, EMS brought us a man directly into Room 4, the trauma room. He came in with complaints of chest pain, SOB (shortness of breath), and a small laceration of the bridge of the nose. The room nurse informed the resident the laceration had to be repaired before the patient was moved into the next room, a medical room. The room resident didn't see the patient for about thirty minutes, at the end of which time the patient was clearly in shock. Listening to the nurse, he repaired the laceration and moved the patient.

When the patient got to Room 6, he immediately sustained a respiratory arrest followed by full cardiac arrest. Resuscitation was unsuccessful, and the patient died. Both the room doctor and the room nurse were disciplined. I don't know if the patient would have been resuscitated had he been seen appropriately; I do know he wasn't the way we had managed the patient.

Two days later (12/16/74), a seventy-four-year-old man seen before (12/14/74) in the ED for chest pain and was discharged by the medical resident, returned in full cardiac arrest.

It never ceases to amaze me how well trained people can fail to use common sense, and fail to remember, above all else, do no harm.

Super ED party 12/19/74
Entry: 12/20/74
Floater: T.

It was the beginning of the Christmas season. The hospital wards were decorated. The ED was decorated. Many wards and departments had their own Christmas parties. The hospital had one for the medical staff at a hall. When we moved to the new hospital, the ED had theirs at a hall off campus. During the season chorales wandered the halls and the lobbies.

On 12/19/74, Screening (the walk in area) was closed until 6:00 p.m. and was turned into a kids' playroom—"don't be surprised if nothing in there works." Families of employees attended. There was dancing and singing and the drinking of alcohol enhanced punch—not much.

On 12/20/74, a second party was held in my office for a smaller group of invitees. My office could only hold three people at once during business hours, and they had to be good friends. As a Doctor once said, "it was so small you had to go out to change your mind." I wasn't there so I couldn't assume any blame or glory. The staff managed, I don't know how, to crowd seventeen people into the room. They were sitting on the two chairs, one desk, and two filing cabinets. The rest were sitting on the floor. There was a large soup kettle filled with alcohol enhanced punch they managed to finish. It was a great party and served to enhance the comradeship of the Department.

Chapter VI
A Pregnant Patient

EMS brought a 34 week gravid (pregnant) woman here with severe LAP (lower abdominal pain) after refusing to take her to Hutzel Hospital, according to the family. On arrival she had bulging membranes. Promptly spontaneous delivery. Viable male infant. Mother's condition post partum good. Baby transferred to Children's Hospital preemie ICU.
Entry: 10/20/74
Floater: W.

Eventually the protocol for EMS handling of pregnant patients was modified so women greater than twenty weeks pregnant were taken to the labor and delivery room of a cooperating and close hospital. Even though we had no delivery or labor rooms, fifty to sixty live births a year were delivered in the ED. On 8/13/81, we had our first live birth at DRH (new hospital).

When a woman in active labor came in, she was taken to the resuscitation room, or quickly checked at Triage. If delivery was impending, we took care of her and the newborn. If not, we tried to transfer her to Hutzel Hospital or Detroit Memorial Hospital, located right across the street from DGH. The transfer to the latter was by gurney pushed fast, across the street.

Virtually all the doctors in the ED traipsed in, as well as the nurses and medical students, followed by a variety of students, housekeepers, and police officers. Both the gynecology and the pediatric residents were called. Sometimes, they even made it in time. But everything was the responsibility of the emergency physicians and nurses assigned to the resuscitation. After birth, the mother was transferred to Hutzel and the baby to Children's. When the pregnant mother arrived, regardless of the method of transportation, she was taken directly into the resuscitation area, and placed on a gurney designed to handle women who required a pelvic examination or delivery. An incubator was moved in as well as the pediatric resuscitation cart, containing pediatric medication and intubation equipment, followed closely by the doctor and nurses assigned to the area. Then everyone else came. After some 5000 years of women delivering their babies in a variety of places, often without a physician in attendance, a crowd was obviously required at a birth in the ED.

I was, and am, amazed at the number of young women who apparently didn't know they were pregnant, or at term. Needless to say, their parents, including their mother, didn't know either. Many did not have prenatal care, and had never seen a doctor, or gone to a clinic. Lots of the mothers continued smoking, drinking alcohol, or taking drugs throughout the pregnancy. It wasn't a race or economic class issue either.

Oh well, it was exciting, invigorating, and made the day that much more pleasant. It was nice to see a healthy baby born. It was not always happiness.

Breech delivery in ER last niter; gyn resident responded (2 calls. Pt. go 1(first pregnancy) BOW (bag of waters) ruptured (2 hrs in ER Delivered about 24 wk. fetus with cyanotic color no onset respiratory efforts. Gyn resident impression was nonviable fetus instructed nurses to cover fetus and place in incubator—a nurse noticed heart rate palpable at apex 60. Resuscitation started by moonlighter. Baby responded or improved CHM responded intubated baby and transfer to CHM. Outlook poor. Raises moral, ethical, medical questions.

Entry: 9/20/77
Floater: TP

I am not sure why TP felt compelled to raise this question. Because I believed that any patient, unless we were instructed differently by a legal device, or the patient himself, was entitled to have an attempt at resuscitation, so was this baby. Our general rule was that any patient who was warm was entitled to an attempt at resuscitation. Including babies. This baby was a peculiar problem. This child had no respiratory efforts and was cyanotic. Resuscitating her may have meant a lifetime as a vegetable or a lifetime with a severe handicap. Breech deliveries in the ER were really tough and it was especially tough to protect the airway when the cord was wrapped around the neck.

My youngest child, my daughter, had been a difficult delivery. I was standing outside the delivery room when she was born. She had no respiratory movements even after the traditional slap. She developed cerebral palsy. When I reread this note, I noticed a subtle change in the words TP used. He went from calling the baby a fetus to a baby.

As I said, not all deliveries were happy. My daughter's was.

Stillborn 5/1/82
Entry; 5/3/82
Floater: Krome
Problem case. Police prisoner, PV, age)75, diagnosed with senile dementia with paranoid features. Patient arrested after he shot 2 police officers. Patient in O.C.U.)48 hours. Psychiatry recommends hospitalization of patient. Exact location depending on whether charges are maintained or dropped by police. Two police officers informed the psychiatrist that a judge would show up to arraign the patient. No judge showed (today). Admission, therefore, at a stalemate.
Entry: 10/31/74
Floater: M

We had lots of emotionally disturbed patients. We had lots of prisoner patients. And a fair number of both. For psychiatric prisoners who required admission for their mental disease there were three choices. If the charges were minor and dropped, they could be sent to a psych institute for treatment, or admitted to our own psych floor. If the charges were not dropped, they were arraigned, and could be court ordered to a state institute, the state hospital for criminally insane. Because they did not require peculiar security arrangement, DRH or a state facility were to be used. Medically ill or injured patients could be admitted to our prisoner ward.

Mentally disturbed patients were the bane of my existence from 1969 until I left in 1984. The first meeting I had in July, 1969, was regarding the handling of mentally disturbed patients. Large volumes of these unfortunate people inundated us every day; many more than our resources could handle. DRH was the crisis center for most of the county and it showed.

Frequently, the psych staff could not keep up with the load. The Crisis Center could be filled with patients, and many others were in the department waiting to be moved into the crisis center. All admissions, at that time, needed a medical history and physical examination, as well as laboratory studies and a chest x-ray. The patients were strapped down to the gurney, so a lot of gurneys were tied up, contributing to our lack of gurneys. Screaming, yelling and swearing, they only added to the chaos.

Many were homeless, alcoholic or substance abuse patients. Many were aggressive or violent. Many were paranoid. Many were suicidal. Sometime in the late seventies, Michigan, in an attempt to save money, cutback on the number of beds at state psych institutes, and then, closed many. Patients were, in theory, to be treated in outpatient facilities close to where they lived. Since many were homeless, arrangements had to be made for some to be housed in half way houses, residential living situations (group homes). It became harder and harder to admit patients, and many simply recycled- state facility —group home —-DRH —-back to the state facility; a never ending cycle.

Some ten to fifteen years later, when I was working in a suburban hospital that also had a number of psychiatric patients, I noticed a significant difference from the urban psych patients. The patients in Detroit tended to be more vocal, more violent and more paranoid. I don't know what accounted for the difference but I am sure there is a social worker someplace who could write a paper about it.

One evening, at about four or five, a court social worker called. A patient committed to NSH (Northville State Hospital) had shown up in court, where the judge released her. When the court closed, the inmate was still sitting in the court room. She had no place to go. So the court worker wanted to return the inmate to us to find her a place to live. The worker wasn't happy when I told her the court social worker should work this out; don't return her to DGH!

Our mentally disturbed patients were restrained with leather straps to the gurney—sometimes all four limbs; sometimes two (a wrist and leg). But if they were really aggressive and violent this didn't stand in their way. Patients escaped by squirming out of restraints or cutting them with a smuggled in knife, or by conning another patient to release them. Sometimes they talked medical students into loosening the restraints. Mostly, restraints were applied to protect the patient, staff, or other patients. From time to time, a new physician thought this was horrible and would release the patient only to have the patient elope, or hit another patient. There were repercussions if the restraints were released.

NL—psych head trauma by another pt. in 8.
Entry: 8/22/78
Floater: BCW
JJ jumped out of 3rd floor window 9-13 while on citation and without restraints and died.
Entry: 9/15/78
Floater: BCW

One Sunday morning, I went into the crisis center to do history and physicals and each patient was singing a different hymn. I called for quiet and told them that although it was all right to sing, everybody had to sing the same hymn. There were a few moments of relative silence while they chose the hymn, Rock of Ages. They all sang the same hymn.

In O.C.U., one day a patient was swearing as loud as he could, disturbing all the medical patients and being generally disruptive. I was called to sedate the patient, not yet seen by psych. The nurse informed me the patient was paranoid and I should be careful.

"What's the problem sir?'

Loud swearing ensued, reflecting on my choice of sexual partners and on my mother.

"Sir, if you keep being noisy and yelling at the nurses, I'll have to report you."

He never yelled again and begged me not to report him. Sometimes you just had to play into their fantasy.

I was conducting a tour for city officials. Lying on a gurney in the hall was a mentally disturbed patient strapped down one on one. He had just quieted down when our group approached. The patient called one of the city councilmen over. As he started to go to the patient's side, I suggested as diplomatically as possible this was not a good idea. The councilman went anyhow. The conversation, paraphrased, went like this:

The councilman shakes hands and introduces himself.

"What can I do for you, sir?"

"Nothing, you mother fucking white honkey prick."

I pulled the councilman back. "I guess I can't count on him to vote for me in the next election!" It must have all worked out alright. The councilman went on to become a senator from Michigan. A damn good one, too.

Chapter VII
Routine Day

Subject: bomb threat. At 11:25 p.m., communications received a bomb threat via telephone by an unknown person directed to Ward 3-3. Bomb was set to go off at 12 MN. Police were notified by ADO, also notified security guard and disaster chief, Dr. L. Apparently call was a hoax as no bomb found and none went off. General security measures were discussed between me and Mr. H (ADO), to the extent such a threat related to Emergency Department.
Addendum: bomb threat
Entry: 11/29/75
Floater: M.

Bomb scares were intermittent but not rare. And when they came, we never found out from where, and whom. The police came and arrangements were made for the potential of evacuating patients. Ambulances were called in just in case. The bomb squad came with search dogs. Nothing was found. For a while they were in vogue, but then they stopped. No bomb ever blew.

Have switched from cuprex to kvell for delousing with a miserable success rate—3 patients last week were not 'cured'.

Big crisis over O2 tanks...
Entry: 12/1/75
Floater: T.

One room was set aside for delousing patients. But ventilation was poor and we had to use fans to limit the toxic fumes which made patients and staff sick. We used the DOA room, but that only had a tub. At the new hospital (DRH), a shower and tub were both installed. Ventilation was improved.

Because we had a large number of homeless patients, who slept on the street, in shelters or in the parks, under bridges or under train trestles; a lot of patients required delousing. A room dedicated to these patients was a necessity and was used often. Some homeless people came in just for the showers—once a month. This was the only bath and shower they ever used. And, of course, for the food and clothes.

After delousing, the patients were given new clothes the volunteers had collected, and fed a 'Kromeburger.' Discharged, they frequently returned to the same setting that gave them lice the first time.

Much of what we did, and the patients we saw, were part of a never-ending cycle.

Big crisis over O2(oxygen) tanks. Only 1 tank (SOS-supplier of portable O2 tanks) left in ED, and the company didn't give any replacements, as the free stuff ran out yesterday. GS's (hospital purchasing agent) office refused to pay them. Anyway after a long discussion, GS OK'd the SOS and they are returning our supply tonight.

It was hard to educate the variety of purchasing officers we had. They rarely understood our needs. We frequently ran out of medication and equipment. Vendors got to the point of not delivering supplies unless the hospital paid in advance, because the hospital was such a notorious poor payer.

Once we ran out of sterile four by fours. The purchasing agent made a stat purchase. He called to tell me that the sponges would be in the next day, and he had gotten a great price. When they arrived, the nursing director and I both understood why the price was so good. The sponges were two inch suqare, and not sterile. Great buy.

All patients then and now have the right to refuse treatment even if it would save their life. We felt, rightly so, that we had an obligation to do what was best for the patient. If the patient was compromised by psychiatric disease or substance abuse, including alcohol, we would seek legal or administrative or medical intervention.

Second major problem Pt. MZ, #801078, with open fracture (Lt) ankle (probe under the influence of ethanol) refused surgery and signed AMA (Against Medical Advice). Efforts are under way to sober her up and apprise her of seriousness of open fracture of ankle. Patient in active state of denial. If patient continues to refuse, I would recommend involvement of administration because if this woman doesn't get fixed and soon she may very well lose part of her leg. If that's the way it goes, we will need plenty of witnesses.

Krome's nb: *"See 12/30/75. Ms. Z's son got himself declared legal guardian and surgery went forward."*

Chapter VIII
Substance Abuse

*Meth (*adone*) patient from north-east clinic wanted Valium as treatment for missed methadone dose—-patient talked to and refused.*
Entry: 9/29/74
Floater: BN

The world has probably never seen a time when substances were not abused. In the late '60s and '70s, drug abuse became an ever increasing problem. In the '60s, it was largely hallucinogens and marijuana, against a backdrop of heroin. As time went on, heroin use became more common, and, then came cocaine in all its forms. But during this same time period, heroin use increased and drug houses and street corner capitalists burgeoned. Against this background, the city, county and surrounding counties all became active in the war on drugs. Even the federal government eventually got involved. Education, rehabilitation, prison, invading other countries, have all been used. The best we have accomplished is a truce.

Methadone became the drug of choice for treating heroin addicts. It wasn't uncommon for addicts to come in and tell us they missed their methadone dose, and asking for some. Each clinic has a twenty-four-hour emergency number on a card the patient was to carry at all times. Many did not carry the card, or "lost" them. Even prisoners on methadone were supposed to get missed doses. Consequently, they were brought to us even though the ER never gave missed doses.

Not all junkies are unemployed street people. Some are employed, well educated, and well off financially, and knew how to control their habit. They might take vacations to get clean and returned to work, and to the drugs. There were auto workers who used drugs while working on the line. In fact, it was a Detroit adage that one never bought a car built on either a Monday or Friday; when workers were just off the weekend or getting ready for the weekend off.

Against this background of substance abuse, drug wars and open trafficking in drugs, the various governments decided something had to be done. Jails were, and are, filling up quickly with abusers, but it wasn't helping and the education push hadn't yet begun in any real strength, not that I am sure it ever worked. Methadone maintenance clinics sprang up for heroin addicts and were financed in a variety of ways.

I had a two-year experience in the service, the Public Health Service, from 1962 through 1964, at the Public Health facility in Lexington, Kentucky. Narco, as it was known, was a minimum security prison and a hospital facility for narcotic, meaning heroin, addicts. Some inmates were there voluntarily; some received federal sentences incarcerating them. All had a history of current or recent heroin addiction. Many bad guys when arrested would tell the judge drugs made them do it. Then wind up being sentenced to Narco.

The clinics in and around Detroit were using methadone for maintenance, based on the philosophy that if you could give junkies a legal medicine, free or low cost, then they would have no reason to commit crimes to get money for drugs. This was, as everyone would find out, a failed philosophy. Many junkies enjoyed the high from heroin, and kept using even when on methadone. Many were denied access to such programs. Many couldn't handle the rigidity of the programs—attendance at group meetings, constant monitoring, etc.

When it became known that I had experience with methadone for detoxification, I was approached, with pressure by our social worker, who felt it was our obligation as city health institution to start a clinic. So we did. The clinic was run out of the ER, with junkies coming in to drop urine samples and pick up methadone. In time, the number of city clinics increased to the point it was no longer necessary for us to continue. After two to three years our travel in this mess was stopped. Thank God. To the best of my memory, we never had a single success. When it was over, the treatment group had bought, or stolen, a trophy to thank me. They held back on giving it until they could get it engraved. I never saw it.

Our group meetings were held once a week, facilitated by our social worker. I even invited three of the group to my house for dinner. They were polite and courteous and said all the appropriate things to my wife and kids. I remember to this day their sitting on the floor playing games with my sons. I almost felt they were "normal." Three weeks later one died from an over dose, and one was stabbed to death on the street.

One worked as a bouncer at a dope house; a nice enough guy and very big. He told me how much he liked me and how he would anything for me. If anyone was giving me trouble, he said, he would break both their knees for only twenty-five dolalrs; half his usual fee. Although I must admit it was a tempting offer, I never took him up on it.

Severe problem

Subject: Narcotics (missing). At morning report today it was reported that 2 doses of morphine sulfate are missing. And 2 doses of Demerol are over the count.

Pharmacy representative up to meet with me and Mrs. L....

It was decided to turn in all ED doses and record sheets on morphine and Demerol.

Further, pharmacy to reissue new doses of above with new sheets so that miscount to previous 24-48 hours.

Mrs. L...was directed to

Obtain statement from charge nurses involved because usual shift change narcotics count was not done between off going and oncoming charge RN's as required.

Ask doctor on ward to obtain urine on one of the patients to assay for morphine if possible. This would help if MS was substituted for Demerol by some chance.
Date: 12/29/75
Floater: JNM

Missing narcotics were not common, but not unusual. There were controls limiting staff ability to access controlled substances. To access the narcotic cabinet, a cabinet locked within a cabinet, a nurse had to have the keys which were passed from the lead nurse to lead nurse. Only they had the keys. The nurse administering the medication took what was needed and signed a log sheet, with the patient's name and number and the dose given, while the lead nurse watched.

A professional staff member caught pilfering drugs, was fired and the licensing board notified; their professional license was lifted. Over time, attitudes became more liberal and the professional, who sought help, prior to being caught, was put into a rehab program and their license suspended. In my naivety, I couldn't believe that nurses and doctors would pilfer drugs for their own use.

But I learned that medical and nursing staff included the same sorts of people that lived on the outside, maybe not as many but the same variety.

During my two years at Narco, I had learned that even "nice people" could be junkies, including doctors and nurses. Most junkies used heroin; the medical professionals used drugs they could access at work—morphine, Demerol, barbiturates, tranquilizers. But they had some personality characteristics in common; ingratiating, gregarious and seeking instant gratification.

Some inmates were there voluntarily; some received federal sentences incarcerating them. I worked for two years on the "shooting gallery," where incoming patients and prisoners were housed until physically clean of heroin. Usually, this took from three to ten days, depending on their addiction. Inmates were given methadone if they showed physical signs of withdrawal; then detoxified from that point with ever decreasing doses until no longer physically dependent. Some had other addictions which treated at the same time. When detoxified, they were released into the general population for up to six weeks of treatment.

Inmates who were volunteers frequently signed out and returned home, to their lives. Some stayed clean; some we saw again the following year—the "vacationers." I hated my job, even though it was not menial and not especially hard work. There was enormous pressure from the inmates for sleeping pills, pain pills, and off duty assignments. When I was discharged from the service, I vowed to never again get involved in with druggies.

There were three categories of admission: prisoners, heroin users sent there for their sentence; volunteers, who came voluntarily to get withdrawn, usually for a vacation period from work; and, "C-vols," coerced by some regulatory agency, or the courts, to come for the cure, until released by us. "C-vols" could be arrested on discharge, or subject to regulatory restrictions. We notified the coercing body when they left prematurely. There were some success stories, although there was a ninety-five perent recidivism rate. I can recall at least once when we managed to get a nurse's license back.

Lots of patients felt uncomfortable, but few had physical signs.

Medical professionals went through a peculiar withdrawal. They expected special treatment, and were unsettled when they didn't get it. It went about like this:

Day 1: My name is Dr. Krome. It is my job to get you through this process. You will be uncomfortable, but you will not have any physical withdrawal. We use methadone. You will get a dose every time you show any signs, physical signs; of withdrawal then you will be detoxified from the methadone, slowly. It shouldn't take more than 5 days, frequently less. Do you have any questions?

Dr. Patient: Do you know I am a doctor?

Krome: Yes, and unless you complete the entire course of therapy, including counseling, we will notify your licensing board, and you'll most likely loose your license. Try and relax and take it one day at a time.

Day 2:
Dr. Patient: I feel terrible and I didn't sleep the whole night.
Krome: We can give you something to help you sleep. According to the nurses, however, you showed no physical signs of withdrawal.
Dr. Patient: I didn't think it would be like this.
Day 3:
Krome: How's it going?
Dr. Patient: I didn't sleep again last night. I feel terrible, and I can't do it.
Krome: Doctor, you are a junkie. You have no choice, unless you don't want your license back. From now until the day you die, you will be a junkie. Accept it. Live with it. Doctor or no doctor, you are a junkie. Go with the program.

Soon after I started at DGH, the head ER nurse and I thought it would be a good idea for our nurses to have an understanding of what is done by nurses in a real ER. So with much finagling we arranged for one of our young nurses to spend a month in Lansing. I called the chief of the ED there, and he, very kindly, suggested she live with him and his family. When she returned she would lecture all three shifts of nurses about what she had learned. All went well. Then about one month after she got back she turned yellow. She had hepatitis and admitted she was a heroin abuser. I called my friend to tell him how his good deed was rewarded. His entire family had to receive medication to attempt to prevent hepatitis. "No good deed ever goes unpunished."

Substance abuse in Detroit like a lot of other cities was and is a large problem. Although, as I said, drugs were a changing scene, heroin remains a constant. The number of abusers, drug and alcohol, with their complications kept us busy. Year after year they kept coming. They made up close to fifteen to twenty percent of our patients.

In the '70s hallucinogens came bursting forward. I don't mean just marijuana, also LSD, peyote, mescaline, and others. Free rock concerts were in, and we provided first aid at them. I was asked by a reporter if our going to give first aid wasn't condoning the use of drugs. He didn't like it when I asked him if his station covering them didn't do the same. But every free concert had drugs all over. Many of the kids were having trips; some good, some bad.

In cooperation with a number of communities around Detroit we started outreach programs; going into the community to talk about drugs with users and parents. There were two of us that did it, gaining a fair amount of good publicity for DGH and the ED. As our notoriety increased, so did the number of users. But an emergency room was probably the worse place for hallucinogen users on a bad trip. That's all they needed, the additional auditory and visual stimuli could keep them in a bad trip. They would scream and yell. The use of tranquilizers might help some; but basically we would try to keep them in a darkened quiet room, until they came down.

We never went a day without an abuser; if not drug, then, alcohol. And when an alcoholic came in intoxicated, they were really drunk. It wasn't rare for us to have them unconscious and with a blood alcohol in the 3-500 (below 100-range was sober) range. There were some so drunk that they required intubation. And there were those who made it to 800 and still lived. Of course, some didn't. There was a 500 club for those who made it to that level and survived. And, of course, there were the complications, including pancreatitis, bleeding, and seizures. The seizures were mostly in those who were withdrawing from alcohol. All intoxicated, or apparently intoxicated, patients had a physical examination and blood drawn. Those with signs of trauma who were difficult to awaken eventually had a head CT. I am not sure, to this day, why we drew blood alcohol levels on the repeaters without trauma. It was, I think, a habit.

There were the junkies; too numerous to count. Many, many heroin overdoses; and other drug overdoses. Waking an unconscious junkie could be a unique experience. Given a narcotic antagonist, they came charging out of their stupor. Frequently, we restrained them before we gave the antagonist.

RG—phencyclidine)24 hours
Entry: 2/14/80
Floater: BCW

Phencyclidine (PCP) was a hallucinogen. This guy had a bad trip. We kept some of them in OCU for a prolonged time. We all knew that the one place someone with a bad trip did not belong in was the ER. It was hard to quiet them down. The best place was a nice quiet room with minimum lighting and someone to talk to them and maintain a semblance of contact with reality.

1 heroin OD extubated
Entry: 5/1/80
Floater: JET

Heroin overdosed patients often ended up intubated (tube placed in airway to help them breath) they were so deeply asleep. Once the antagonist was given sometimes repeatedly, they woke up and could be extubated. When they came in and were breathing poorly, they went to the resuscitation room as a code. Lots of people responded; someone intubating the patient and others trying to start an IV; a difficult task in a drug addict who had used his veins up. If we were smart, he was physically restrained to the gurney before given a narcotic antagonist. Once given this, the patient would sit bolt upright screaming. His pupils became dilated; he started breathing.

(KS) 24 hours DT's OCU
Entry: 5/7/80
Floater: BFB

DT's (delirium tremens) were usually treated in the ED. Most could be broken during that time. Some developed a temperature elevation and pneumonia and had to be admitted. Others took longer to break. DT'er's were common. They had IV's started and were given mild sedation. All had lab studies and chest x-rays taken. Those with pneumonia were admitted. At one time the mortality rate for DT's was thirty percent. But this wasn't the case at DGH/DRH.

As a surgery resident I was given the task of reviewing our post operative complications. Far and away, was DT's.

There is no segment of society immune from the substance abuse syndrome. I already told the story of one of our nurses who caught it. When I was in the service I met the rich and famous who also fell to this disease. At Narco, each Friday at lunch time the inmates would put on a concert. It was fantastic, and I met a number of musicians who were in the Playboy Jazz Hall of Fame. Even today the media is filled with stories of substance abusers. I had hired one doctor who was in a rehabilitation program, and years later another physician had his license lifted and was arrested for continual drunk driving. His promising career over, his family destroyed, and his "friends" had abandoned him. Our government has poured millions of dollars into the effort to stem this tide.

There is one sadder, very sad story to tell in this arena.

Even before I took my job, I had made it a prerequisite that I have a secretary. The city, working as it usually did, didn't get me one for some time. Until then I had to borrow secretarial time from others—-either in the Department of Surgery or in hospital administration. Those secretaries had other primary responsibilities, which limited the time they could give to me. There was no one to answer the telephones or file or do the mail, other than me. So I spent a lot of time doing things that had little to do with my responsibilities; sort of the work plan for my future here.

One day, an administrator brought a young lady to my office, and introduced her as my secretary. We talked for a few minutes, and I found out she had just graduated from high school and this was her first full time job. When she asked me when she could start, I said now and sat her at my desk. Orientation would occur as time progressed, but right now she could start by answering the telephone.

Over time, she ran the office and my professional life. She was empowered to make my appointments, arrange my travel, do typing and filing. She became, in essence the departmental secretary. She took care of the medical students, the residents, the contract doctors. I cannot begin to tell you all the things she did. She was the focal point of our EMT training program. All the students knew her; all the residents knew her, all the people who had any contact with the department knew her. But even with this she had an outside social life as any teenager would have; she even got two of her friends jobs at the hospital. She had a boyfriend and went to the free rock concerts. When I got active in national organizations, she began doing that work too. Although she lived at home with her mother, eventually she moved into her own apartment. She even went to a national meeting with my wife and me, at no expense to her.

Over the years we got closer, as she did with everyone in the department. She went to dinners with staff and with residents. She came to my house and to others. She baby sat for some of the staff. In short, she became an integral part of us, professionally and socially. She was like a daughter to me, and I really cared about her.

Her work environment and her social pressure from those around her at work put enormous pressure on her. I know that now. I didn't realize it at the time.

Maybe this explains it. None of us were looking for anything. She was so integral to us, we worked on the assumption she was like us in the sense of sharing our morals and ethics. She didn't, but we didn't know it for a long time.

As time went on, she stopped doing the boring things around the office, like filling. Her typing fell behind. She took long lunch hours and breaks. She even started taking breaks to catch a nap. Once she fell asleep at her desk. Few people saw this. I did, but I ignored the obvious. We used to keep some petty cash in the drawer in my desk. Gone. Samples of Valium were also kept there. Gone. Eventually it became obvious that she was on the nod. I confronted her and told her she had to go into rehabilitation or lose her job. She went into rehab. But it failed and she came out addicted. She was taking methadone, heroin, and stealing Valium from our staff. She got thrombophlebitis of her leg, and hepatitis. She was hospitalized in various hospitals. She took more and more sick time and personal time. Her vacation time was gone; personal time, gone; sick time, gone. Medical staff told me to do something; she was making a bad impression for the department. And my not getting rid of her wasn't helping.

When I left to go Beaumont, I didn't take her. She became very depressed and either committed suicide or died from infection. Lots of people came to the funeral which was very sad and depressing. Another young victim of the substance abuse war.

Chapter IX
No Entry

The patient incident
No entry
Floater: B.

It was a warm summer day, the kind that is, in emergency medicine, usually associated with increased interpersonal violence. I don't remember the exact date. I was in East Lansing, Michigan, for an all day meeting of some committee. Someone passed me a message that I was to call the floater as soon as possible. B. would not call me for any trivial matter, so I knew it was important. I broke from the meeting, went to my room and called. When he got on the phone, I could tell from his tone something was seriously wrong.

How is it going, Ron?
Boring but OK. Is something wrong?
I don't know how to tell you this.
Is my wife ok?
Yeah
Is your wife ok?
Yeah

Are my kids ok?
Yeah
Your kids?
Yeah
It sounds as though anything you have to tell me doesn't involve those close to us, so just let it out.
Ok. Your right. Here it is. One of your nurses just stabbed and killed a patient.

I was stunned and sat down on the bed. I couldn't think of anything to say. Finally, I continued.

Tell me again but slower so I can absorb it.
One of your nurses went and got a scalpel and slit a patient's throat. She died in the OR. So did her unborn baby.

Now, I was really dumbfounded. I had noticed he kept referring to the nurse as one of "my nurses." Usually, they were our nurses. I guess it was like kids. When they were good, they were their mother's; when they were bad, they were their fathers. Although I had only been in my job for a few short years, I had talked to other people across the country that had jobs similar to mine. None of them had ever told me of an incident such as this.

Ron? Are you still there?
Yes. Have the police been notified?
She has been arrested.
Ok. Now we have to take some steps that you can start until I get there.
Suspend her immediately, with pay pending investigation.
Notify the personnel officer of what happened and what we have done.
Next, notify the director of the hospital yourself. Don't rely on anyone else to do it.
Get written statements from everyone who saw or heard anything. If the police are already doing it, tell them you need copies for us.

Make sure the nursing supervisor knows everything we have done and what has happened. Prepare a summary of events, and everything you know for sure happened, don't put any opinions on paper. I'll be there in an hour or so and meet you at the hospital.

When I got there I reviewed his summary, the statements, and talked to him. Then I called the personnel officer and hospital director. Neither wanted us to do anything else. We meet with the nursing staff and allowed them to ventilate. They were especially angered because none of the hospital security personnel were available or came to the scene. They were all defensive of the nurse.

According to my memory as near as I can piece together, this is what happened. The nurse, an LPN (Licensed Practical Nurse) was working in Screening. It had its own small waiting room. One doctor and one nurse was all the manpower assigned. Screening was a high volume, high turnover area.

The visitor, in the waiting area, took great umbrage because she had to wait. Each time the nurse came out to call somebody in, the visitor, literally got in her face and increased her vitriolic harangue not making the nurse very happy. As time passed, and the discussion passed through all the stages of anger, no one called for help from the nursing supervisor, the floater, or the screening doctor; any of whom might have calmed them both and resolved the conflict. Security personnel were not in the area. Although, even today I am not sure how much help they would have been.

The nurse left Screening and went to the treatment areas, where the scalpels were kept, and took one. When she got back, the visitor once again raised her rhetoric up several thousand decibels. At this point, the nurse warned the visitor to back off. She didn't. The nurse opened the scalpel and slit the visitor's throat. As we found out later, it was a highly significant slash, cutting both carotid arteries and the jugular vein. The visitor and her unborn child died on the operating room table.

Two years later, the nurse was found not guilty because the act was considered self defense. She was returned to full status with two year's back pay. When the personnel officer told me she would be back in the ER, I told him that only one of us will show up. If she did I would turn around and leave. She didn't come back.

The Shooting Incident

I was, once again, out of town when it happened. I was on the west side of Michigan at another "have to" meeting. It was the summer of 1971, hot even for Michigan; the kind of hot that makes people do strange things. When I got back I heard about it, the whole hospital was talking about it. The stench of the tear gas permeated the entire ED although it was three days since it all came down. As near as I can remember, the shooting and killing went about like this.

There was a social worker, a woman, who worked in the ED, and who had been of enormous help in setting up our methadone clinic. In fact, she ran the weekly group meetings, a requirement for all our junkies. She was a pleasant, hard working lady, rather attractive but not a raving beauty. She related well to virtually all hospital employees, and, to the best of my knowledge, was never accused of bigotry of any type, a unique reputation at DGH. She dated black and white men. She was white.

There was the clerk; an angry young man under the best of circumstances. He worked in the ED, registering patients. Sometimes there would be a confrontation; nothing physical; but, sometimes loud and aggressive. To the best of my recollection he had never been disciplined for anything major. He was black.

The clerk and the social worker had dated. The social worker claimed that the clerk had raped her. When she told me the story later, I believed her. But she never made out a police report, never been examined. She told her story to the assistant director of the hospital, who had an affinity for her; he looked at her as his daughter.

Anyhow, he believed her. But since there was no police report or physical examination, there was no hard evidence. But he fired the

73

clerk. The clerk had gone through the union grievance procedure, and still lost. Now we come to the summer, with the heat, and a pissed off employee. It was early in the afternoon; the sun was summer bright, no inkling of rain, no shade, although it would cool some as the sun went down.

He walked up the stairs in the front of the hospital, through the front door, into the main lobby. He wore a shirt and tie, and a jacket. Along his side, in one hand, he carried a rifle. He went through the main lobby, came out the other side. He took a right turn, down a short hall, to the administrative suite. He entered the suite. No on stopped him or approached him. It was about a three minute walk, all the time carrying his rifle in plain view. He went into the administrative suite.

On his left, as he entered, was an office. In it sat an administrative assistant, the controller of the hospital. He was nice, well liked man, with a young family. The clerk went straight into the secretaries' office. To his left was the assistant director's office and to his right, the office of the director. Both were empty. He asked for the assistant director by name, raising his rifle. The secretary said he wasn't in; would he like to talk to someone else? There were two secretaries in the office and the wife of the chief of surgery. When they saw the rifle they went under the desks. But not before he got one shot off and hit a secretary in the arm, breaking both bones in her forearm. The people in the office buried themselves deeper under the desks, terrorized. Mr. AA came in from his office and caught one in his chest, slumped back against a wall where he would be found later.

The police had been called; they surrounded the office. The office was located in a corner of the hospital on the first floor. The police surrounded the outside and entered the hospital. They didn't want to rush the office, afraid that the others would be killed. It was a real hostage situation. The streets were blocked off; the first floor evacuated. The clerk was shooting out the windows. The police returned fire. Tear gas was lobbed in, and the office became quiet. Surgeons were called from the OR.

The police rushed in, got the others out of the office and into the ED. The tear gas was thick and everyone suffered from inhalation.

They found the clerk dead; Mr. AA was bleeding from his chest, slumped against the wall; hardly breathing. He was wheeled down to the resuscitation room in the ED; a cloud of tear gas following him. The surgeons attempt to resuscitate him failed; impeded by the tear gas and the tear gas masks covering their faces.

So ended the famous shooting incident; two dead, including the shooter; two terrorized women who would carry this incident with them for years; a shot secretary, who's arm would take years of rehab to come back, one young family destroyed; and a social worker with a cloud over her for years; a man who would have trouble living down what he had done to a clerk. Finally, at the funeral for the clerk, there was a large turnout of employees. At the funeral for Mr. AA, there was also a crowd. The incident and those involved would not be soon forgotten.

Chapter X
Patient P.

Patient P. brought in 7/24/74 as down and out seen and transferred to social services as OBS (organic brain syndrome) for placement....
Entry 7/25/74
Floater: T.

Patients who were "down and out" were homeless, confused, and who had no significant medical problems. "OBS," was a medical problem which was generally felt, at that time, to be associated with increasing confusion, no significant psychiatric problem, and no overwhelming medical problems. Today it would be called' "Alzheimer's disease." They had to be seen by the room physician, have a chest x-ray, to make sure there was no tuberculosis (Tuberculosis was endemic in Detroit). And some routine laboratory studies, and referred to social work for placement, which could be to a group home or a basic nursing home. Homeless people who were not confused could be sent to a shelter. Of course, this presumed that the evaluation failed to detect any significant treatable medical problem.

The social worker who saw P. thought the patient was more confused than he should be and took it upon himself to order a skull x-ray. There was no such thing as CAT scans. The skull x-ray showed a fracture and the patient was hospitalized for observation.

This social worker had been with us for years and he would be for years to come. He was a sharp, knowledgeable, caring and diligent man. But he was a child of the sixties, a flower child, with long hair-often in a single pigtail—and a mustache, who dressed down. He was known to take an occasional drink and a joint when not at work. He never came to work high. To this time he had picked up, on his own, a cervical spine fracture, two subdural hematomas, and, at least two skull fractures. He saved the patients and us a lot of grief.

These were the days which required a high clinical acumen and judgment of the doctors. Of those things high on the list of technologic advances, that changed the practice of emergency medicine, CT scans were the highest or second highest. In fact, we were only at the stage of using peritoneal taps (a procedure where a needle on a syringe was poked into the abdomen) for the diagnosis of intra-abdominal injuries. Patients with head injuries of any significant degree were admitted for twenty-four hours of observation. Those who got worse or patients with significant neurological signs had arteriography, a procedure with numerous complications, including death. Patients considered to have an intra-abdominal injury had an exploratory laporotomy, a peritoneal tap, or a peritoneal lavage or were admitted for observation. Later, everything was scanned, whether it was necessary or not.

All physicians reported for duty on time.
Entry: 7/28/74
Floater: T.

One could ask why this rates an entry in the floaters log. In fact, there were multiple entries which indicated the presence of staff, medical and nursing. All too frequently we were short staffed until 1976. After that, we hired only full timers, and only those who had completed training in a related specialty. In 1976, we started our own residency in emergency medicine, and didn't feel it was appropriate to have doctors less trained than our residents charged with the responsibility of supervising them.

We used mostly moonlighters. Needless to say, because of our medical staff shortage we were indebted, and dependent on them. They were mostly residents with other full time jobs at the hospital. Some were on-call for their primary service the same night they worked in the ER. I wasn't supposed to know. They weren't allowed to leave the ER when working; but they did.

Their charts were reviewed on a somewhat regular basis. Policy was difficult to enforce or even communicate. Schedules and memos were mailed out to them, but they often denied seeing either. Many were late for their shifts; many, left early, before being relieved. All submitted applications. All were talked to by one of us. The care they rendered was sporadic at best; others were excellent—diligent, hard working and smart. They worked slowly, creating backups.

We only had, at various times, somewhere between one and five full timers. We started with one and eventually went to five; not enough to cover 24/7/365. Even then, they weren't as good as they would become. Certainly, they didn't function as well as contemporary emergency physicians. Neither did I. But we all did the best we could, given the circumstances and the time.

Patients who were hospitalized required lots of nursing care, stressing an already short and very stressed out group. Most were put into the O.C.U. (Observation Care Unit), along with the psychiatric patients waiting for decisions. Patients were supposed to stay no more than twenty-four hours. Few meet this requirement. Here is a list of those waiting longer than twenty-four hours on 7/28/74.

Patient G.—awaiting psychiatry and internal medicine—arrived 7/27/74, 1:05 PM. Diagnosis-psychiatrically disturbed; hypoglycemia

Patient O.—psychiatry and internal medicine—-arrived 7/26/74...Diagnosis-uncontrolled diabetes

Patient L.—awaiting medical resident—arrived 7/26/74 9:19 PM

O.C.U. closed at 3:30 PM because of shortage of staff.
Room 1 closed all day.

Chapter XI
Child Abuse

*Wrong patient sent to...... *
Entry: 10/07/75
Floater: Krome

The wrong psychiatric patient was sent to NSH (Northville State Hospital), a state mental hospital to which we sent patients for hospitalization, always by ambulance. The ambulance attendants failed to check the patient's identification bracelet. Neither did the nursing staff

We didn't always have ID bracelets, and in those times, before ID bracelets, the wrong patient was sometimes moved on down the line. During this pre-historic period, sometimes the wrong name was attached to a patient's remains when they were sent to the morgue, which was not only embarrassing but difficult to explain. There were occasions when an improperly identified body was sent to a funeral home. Needless to say, on these occasions, the family went nuts. Funeral directors weren't too happy either.

Intoxicated and unconscious patients couldn't identify themselves. I am sure, although I never heard of it myself; the wrong patient even received medications not meant for him. There were no ID bracelets for the nurses to use in identifying the patient. Bad times for everyone.

Problems with husband/wife team. 2/yo child problem with 'Protective Services' and DPD. Mother retarded and DT's. Father DT's. (Delirium tremens—an alcohol withdrawal syndrome). Mother took kid home
Entry: 10/08/75
Floater: Krome

The first time I ever saw child abuse was in 1969. Some things you just don't forget; I won't forget this one. I was in my office one evening when one of our administrative personnel called me to see a case in the pediatric section. Sitting up on an examining table was a twelve-year-old boy. Standing next to him was his mother. The boy's shirt was off and lying on the table. Mr. Administrator introduced me and asked the boy to show me his back. It was covered with multiple stripes, long and all running in one direction, from the right lower back straight up to the left shoulder. There was no blood; just long, red, welts. He had been whipped with an electric cord.

I turned to the mother and asked her what happened.

I came home and found him like this.
Ma'am someone beat him. Who?
I don't know.
Who lives with you?
I have a live-in boyfriend. He is the boy's father. He drinks. Did he beat him?
He was drinking and beat him with an electrical extension cord.
Has he done this before?
Yes.
Have you ever notified the police?
Yes. They came over, told my boyfriend if it happened again they would arrest him. When they left, he beat me.

I knew that morally and ethically I was obligated to report this incident. Mr. Administrator and I walked out to talk.

Krome: We have to report it.

Mr. Administrator: If we do, he will beat the hell out of her and him. Then there will be two victims.

Krome: I can't just let it ride, even though I recognize what you are saying.

Mr. Administrator: Try talking to her.

We went back to talk to the mom. I told her what her boyfriend did was cruel and against the law. Her son was at risk to be killed. She listened patiently. Never asking a question. Said she would do what she could to stop it. I told her if her son ever came in like this again, I would get the police involved. She took her son home. I never saw him again. I don't know to this day if he lived or died. I don't know if what I did was right or wrong. All I know for sure is this is some twenty-five years later and it is still on my mind.

This might have been the first case of child abuse I ever saw, it wasn't the last. I had never seen a case in medical school or during my residency. But I saw a lot more over time. Different forms; same result.

They were maimed; burned; had broken bones; forced to drink poisons. There was the "shaken baby syndrome." There were teenagers who had babies; children having children. Unable to take care of the babies they had; sort of unintentional abuse. Generation of unwed mothers living in the same house.

In time, Michigan and our county changed the laws and instituted some real child protection laws. Teachers, doctors, nurses, were obligated to report child abuse to child protective services just on the basis of suspicion. In time, domestic abuse, geriatric abuse, nursing home abuse all achieved national prominence. And more and more cases were reported by suspicious emergency personnel.

2 psych patients gone ran away
Entry: 10/09/75
Floater: Krome

I never really understood how this could happen. In the list of things that seemed to, forever, escape my understanding this was high; along with child abuse, elder abuse, why there isn't peace in the Middle East, why so many children die from starvation each year.

Nursing staff were supposed to be in every area where there were patients. Every psych patient was physically restrained with leather straps——one arm and one opposite leg. Still they managed to escape (go AWOL was the term—Absent Without Leave). Go figure. Sometimes the patients' restraints were cut by another patients, or loosened by a well meaning medical student, or a physician.

Total body burn in
Entry: 10/10/75
Floater: Krome

Young man, trapped in a house fire. House burnt to the ground. He was trapped inside. Brought in by EMS, he was taken directly into the Shock/Resuscitation Room. He actually had a ninety-eight percent body burn, almost all full and partial thickness, as well as smoke inhalation. Only the soles of his feet were not burned. He should have been dead. One doc stood at the head of the bed and intubated him. Two others started IV's using venous cut downs; one at the ankle. The other, in the left subclavian vein, considered a dangerous procedure at that time. Fluids were run in rapidly, labs drawn; portable chest x-rays done; Foley catheter inserted; antibiotics started; tetanus given. Pain medicine given and he was sedated. The dead skin was debrided. He was admitted to the burn unit after getting a whirlpool bath for further debridement.

For two years he was tortured with multiple surgeries; skin debridements, plastic surgery, skin grafts, some using pig skin; some, donated skin from family. He had no skin of his own to use. Multiple whirlpool baths, a special bed, frequent changes of IV's, ventilation assistance. Unable to eat, he had a feeding tube inserted. Slowly, very slowly, he made progress; the intubation tube was converted to a tracheostomy tube. He was slowly weaned to no tube (breathing on his own). The feeding tube was removed. He took oral fluids, then a soft diet, then a regular diet. The IV's were stopped. The antibiotics stopped. The Foley catheter removed. He began walking, first to his chair, then around his room; then around the unit. Finally down the hall. Then he rode down to the hospital entrance in a wheel chair, walked down the steps into a waiting car, and home. He had managed to survive two years, and a horrendous burn. There must be a supernatural force protecting him. He was supposed to have died. Someone had acted on his behalf.

Chapter XII
Mystery Lunches

3) Medical Social worker (HV) on duty 1/5/76, saw patient PB, #860832, but did not make final disposition. Spoke to her at 10 am and at 4 pm disposition had not been made. Patient has been here since 1/3/76 so this odyssey will have to continue tomorrow.
    Entry: 01/06/76
    Floater: B

This patient was still in O.C.U. on 1/7/76. Three days laying on a gurney with a three-inch foam rubber mattress, being taken to the bathroom and eating Kromeburgers. All because the social worker couldn't, or wouldn't, get it done before four p.m.! Unbelievable. We were so inhumane and had such a low level of compassion. Some people just managed to propagate the myth of being a civil service employee, always watching the clock, never missing a break or lunch.

ED lunches arrived on trays in normal fashion. However, the milk cartons were covered with feces which had rubbed off on trays. Sent them back and informed Dietary Supervisor.
    Addendum to #1. Second load of lunch trays brought up and upon inspection were found to have feces on milk, sandwich

wrappers, and disposable tray covers. Called dietary supervisor up to see this and asked her to throw out sandwiches and bring up a clean load. She did this.
Entry: 1/10/76
Floater: B.

To the best of my knowledge, the mystery of the sandwiches was never solved.

B. was the floater when the tray of "shitty" lunches came up, both times. He couldn't believe it and called dietary supervisor to come see. And again when the second tray arrived. We never figured out who did it.

But it did remind me of an incident that occurred when I was an intern, also involving dietary. The house officers and the medical staff ate in the cafeteria. It wasn't unusual for us to find insects swimming in our soup. Finally, one of my colleagues couldn't take it anymore. So he reported, anonymously, the additions to our food to the health department. The cafeteria was closed for three days. No one ever solved, until now, the mystery informant.

GC (gonorrhea) controversy—nobody knows where prisoners with GC should go. HKH wants prisoners seen here. I feel they should extend their philosophy of treatment to everyone, and that includes prisoners.
Entry: 1/12/76
Floater: T.

HKH (Herman Kiefer Hospital) was another city hospital. Originally, it was designed to treat patients with communicable diseases—tuberculosis, meningitis, chicken pox, polio, measles, etc. Polio was so common in those days, that DGH even had a lung respirator. I rotated there for four months as a part of my surgical training, to gain experience with chest surgery. Tuberculosis was treated with drugs and surgery. Sometimes surgery was, at times, a necessity.

HKH ran a venereal disease clinic that treated anyone with suspected sexually transmitted disease (as venereal diseases came to be known). They, as part of the health department, were responsible for tracking all contacts, and encouraging them to get treatment. In the '60s and the early '70s, if a patient presented to our ED with complaints that suggested a STD, he or she, were referred to HKH, VD clinic (euphemistically called the Social Hygiene clinic). In time we started treating patients with STD, and those with positive cultures, were reported to the health department to begin their investigation of known contacts.

There was little herpes and AIDS around, but as time progressed both came to forefront; but not to the exclusion of gonorrhea, chlamydia, or syphilis. Patients were treated according to CDC (Center for Disease Control) guidelines. In the summer of 2004, I picked up three new cases of primary syphilis.

Why we continue to see so much STD remains beyond me. These are diseases which are largely preventable. Everyone knows about condoms. People are taught about the prevention of sexually transmitted diseases in school. When I see a man, or woman, with STD, I can't resist commenting on the use of condoms. But neither can the two nurses who I frequently work with, who often threaten to tell the patient's mother should this recur.

There are a large number of condoms in Detroit that are defective, since, according to my patients they break with an alarming frequency. Maybe CDC needs to study the problem. When I get a patient with their second case of STD, not unusual, I test for syphilis, and suggest they be tested for HIV, something they must do voluntarily.

After the AIDS epidemic started, I had a homosexual man with gonorrhea. I couldn't believe it; this man was a member of the group that brought safe sex to the forefront of the news. The patient appeared to be an intelligent, financially stable man. I couldn't resist telling him how unimpressed I was with his lack of compassion for others. I was livid and it showed. I told him, that if it was up to me, I wouldn't even treat him.

The AIDS epidemic brought its own set of problems. Although we could ask the patient if he had it or was tested for it, we couldn't test for it without the patient's specific approval. In addition, if tested for it in our lab, we couldn't access the results on the computer. Eventually the law was changed so that is a first responder; paramedic or other healthcare provider was exposed to the blood of an AIDS victim the patient could be tested without his specific approval. The results were reported to the medical person responsible for the healthcare provider. Eventually, a rapid test was developed, and treatment could be instituted for the provider within a two-hour window of the exposure. The provider was faced with the problem of safe sex, fear and anxiety. I got hepatitis when I was a senior surgical resident. I wasn't alone. But I never thought I might die from it. Some of my colleagues got tuberculosis, but never thought they would die. Now healthcare workers had to be concerned with living, not just getting sick, and infecting their partners.

You know as I think about it, I realize that if there was no tobacco, alcohol in excess or unprotected sex, ED's around the country could probably close.

The request by Southfield's Providence Hospital asking permission to send their paramedics here for observation in our ED was discussed. Dr. M...agreed to set up and monitor this request with Providence Hospital. Schedule to be sent to Dr. Krome.
Entry: 01/19/76
Floater: JNM

We had EMT (Emergency Medical Technician) training program under the direction of Dr. M...The program was strong and had attained a good reputation for education and training, and was well known around the state. It was under the auspices of Wayne County Community College, and candidates could obtain an AA (Associate of Arts) degree. Students, some of whom were functionally illiterate, were tested and received remedial reading and writing when indicated.

So it wasn't an unusual circumstance for us to get such a request. Already National Guard units and reserve units came to us for additional training and to observe our handling of trauma patients. Our Departmental reputation was growing.

Time was passing and you didn't need much vision to see the future. This was especially true in pre-hospital care. Parts of the country had already progressed to the point of instituting paramedic programs. Southfield, Michigan, was one of these communities. It is just north of Detroit. Dr. M., however, was not in favor moving into this arena. And then there was the problem of money; Detroit didn't have enough to put paramedics on the street. It was hard for us to even increase our EMT numbers. It was a shame. Certainly, the city deserved better care. Second, our Department lost a chance to be a leader in the field.

As a part of running EMS, under state mandate, an EMS Advisory board was formed. Charged with the responsibility of adopting and approving medical procedures, it was, at that time composed of the directors of all five of the city's leading ED's. I was chairman, but everything was done with majority vote. It eventually became obvious that we had too few EMT's to operate a full EMS system. After discussing this with the chief, we elected to notify the mayor, Coleman Young, that more manpower was needed, in a very diplomatic letter. Mr. Young was not happy, he informed us that manpower and other budget issues were not our concern.

5. Dr. B's course in full swing as of today
Entry: 1/26/76
Floater: JNM

Not only were we making progress with pre-hospital care but also with education for practicing emergency physicians. There were only a limited number of residencies in emergency medicine. The largest number of practitioners came from those who had changed from another specialty—second career physicians. Our Department made a commitment to educate and train this pool. Dr. B. developed and put in place a course specifically for second career emergency physicians.

It was a five day course, with animal labs, and other special and independent study courses; with about eight hours a day of educational content. Dr. B. monitored and conducted the course with presentations made mostly by Wayne State faculty. The course, PICEP, ran four times a year. I can't remember the total number of students who took the course, but it was a lot.

The course became so well known and respected, we were invited to put it on at the American College of Emergency Physician's annual meeting. We condensed the course, running it only 9 hours at a time, and repeated it three times. When we were in Dallas, Texas, and put on the course, the College leadership decided we should dine wherever we wanted on them. So, B. and I and his wife, who assisted us went to a very fancy hotel for dinner. I am not sure of the name now, but the dinner was served on fancy plates with fancy linen and fancy utensils. After the appetizer was cleared, the fancy waiter served us sherbet. Now none of us ever having eaten such a fancy meal knew what it was about. Brooks looked at me and I at him. "Did you order desert?" One of us had to ask the waiter, who told us it was a sorbet to clear our pallets. Talk about two rednecks from the backcountry!

M...w...called at 4PM stating he couldn't come to work—his shift was 7PM-7AM—because his car was stuck in the snow—all week. I didn't think that was a valid excuse and told him if he or a replacement didn't show he would be fired
Entry: 2/8/76
Floater: T.

He didn't; he was.

Moonlighters were a problem

When knowledge and performance was really bad we notified their residency director. Even though we weren't required to document the reasons for terminating the employment of a moonlighter, we usually did. One time we had terminated a moonlighter who was a urology resident. When his residency director decided not to renew his contract, for other reasons, he came to us for documentation.

Chapter XIII
Patients

At times I remember things not necessarily stimulated by the entry itself; sort of a spontaneous discharge of memory neurons, not otherwise engaged, sitting quietly in my memory centers. I let my memory flow as I remember; I hope, patients not necessarily covered by the Floater's Log. I can't use people's real names. They have been changed to protect the innocent, the guilty, and the author. Nor are they necessarily in chronological order. My memories do not occur in chronological order, just when there is a spontaneous discharge of the appropriate neurons. As I get older, my memory centers work only spontaneously and never predictably.

The Old Lady on 7

When I was an intern, I had a patient on the seventh floor. She was a sweet old lady, over eighty, with thyroid disease. She had gray hair and wore glasses down on the tip of her nose; the personification of a grandmother. Her religious beliefs were fundamental, to say the least. She was black and a Baptist.

We had ordered her to be given thyroid medications just that day when I was called by the ward nurse that she was refusing to take any medications unless instructed otherwise by God. I went into her room and she told me the same thing. At the nursing station, the nurses and I huddled to plan an alternative. We knew the instructions from God had to come directly from Him (or Her?). not having a communication method with anybody supernatural, we finally decided that the doctor (me) had to handle the situation, since all doctors thought they were gods anyhow. So I wrote out prescription with the patient's name on it. The prescription told her she was to take all the medicines given her by the doctor; I signed it "God." I didn't think that in this case God would mind me forging His name.

Bob

Bob was with us for about seventeen years, arriving, according to my sources, in 1981, and dying in 1998. He was a tall, very light skinned black man, of average weight. People claimed he was the product of a mixed race relationship. He had an engineering degree and had held a nice white collar job until his psychosis took over and he plunged into his own personal Hell. Bob usually wore a suit jacket and a tie. He was a very aggressive and angry psychotic, using more expletives than I'd ever heard coming from *any* one person's mouth. Bob was an active alcoholic and a cocaine abuser.

Bob had a unique ability to stimulate an angry and hostile response from others; doctors, nurses, aides, security personnel, police and paramedics. He really could piss people off for no good reason. Bob had a long history of congestive heart failure and cocaine abuse, but his visits most usually involved trauma. Often he was mugged and there were times he got into a physical altercation even with the police or the paramedics. Someone even broke his arm when trying to restrain him.

One afternoon at the end of the day shift, he cornered me in the write up area. He had a run-in with the nurse in his treatment room, and came to me. Bob: "Dr. Krome, that white, honky bitch has an attitude." All the while, she was writing up his discharge papers, and Bob was standing there tucking in his shirt. She started to tell me what happened; I cut her off; looked at the clock. It was 3:30, and she should have left a half hour ago. I took the discharge papers from her, looked her in the eye, and said, "Punch out and go home." I winked at her. "OK, "she said. And left. Bob looked at me aghast. He told me how pleased he was that I had stood up for him. The nurse, of course, came back the next day.

He had a list of home phone numbers of key people in our administration. One night I got a call from my boss, asking me what was going on with Bob. I told him and asked, "How do you know he is even here? Why are you calling this time of night?"

"Oh, he called me at home." I couldn't believe he had the Boss's home phone number. He even called the vice-president of the hospital at home. How he ever got all these home phone numbers remains a mystery to me to this day.

In 1998, he was taken by an EMS Unit to another hospital, where he died.

Danny

Junkies are unique. They are better at their game than we are at their game. They are con artists. Most are gregarious and ingratiating, and demand instant gratification. A perfect example was Danny. He was a junkie who managed to make the best of his situation, in his mind. I don't know if he is still alive, but he sure permeated my professional life.

Danny was in his twenties when he got shot in the back during a robbery. The gunshot hit his spine and left him a paraplegic. Not a happy situation for anyone. He managed to get state and federal support. Danny went into rehabilitation, learned to live alone and use a wheelchair. For money, he continued to sell drugs, and did very well at it. Tax free, of course. He had enough money for most people to live on, but not enough for him to live in the style to which he would like to become accustomed. He did have enough for the usual jewelry accessories on his neck, wrist, and fingers.

His big problem wasn't his drug habit; he managed that very well. What he didn't manage was his own care. Eventually his butt broke down and he developed decubitus ulcers (pressure sores); big ones that continued to grow, despite visits to the plastic surgery clinic and to the ED. A couple of times he became septic and had to be hospitalized. Danny refused to follow doctor's orders. It just wasn't in him to do the mundane tasks required for the ulcers to heal. So it went: drug abuse, decubitus ulcers, visits to the clinic and hospitalizations. For years.

Eventually, he was admitted for flaps (a layer of skin, and fat to cover his ulcers). The decubitus were covered and the ball was back in Danny's court. He had to take care of the flaps. That failed and over time, despite many visits to the ED, and antibiotics, and pain medicine, the flaps broke down again.

It was time for extreme measures. Danny was septic again. The plastic surgeons had decided to offer Danny extreme surgery. They proposed removing what was left of his legs at the hips. They were useless to him anyhow, went their argument. Removing the legs at the hips left the opportunity to use the tissue from the thighs—skin, fat and muscle—as flaps to cover his decubitus. Danny agreed. So the surgery was done, and both his legs were removed and the flaps swung. They took. Danny had to get off his butt, or the flaps would break down again.

A special gurney was obtained for him; one designed for paraplegics, with big front wheels, so he could lie on his stomach and wheel himself around. Once when he was in the ED, in the OCU, I saw him walking on his hands into the unit, completely nude. He was doing ok.

DC here for 5 days in OCU no one will take him
Entry: 1/7/81
Floater: Krome

That's the story of Danny's life—no one will take him. He had already been thrown out of a number of nursing homes, and the like.

One day, I was reading the morning paper—the Free Press——one of my favorite columnists, and there was Danny's name. This columnist came across Danny lying on his new gurney in front of the old Hudson's building; a busy area in downtown Detroit. In front of him was a sign that said he was a 'Nam veteran and had received his injuries in that war. He told the columnist that he was unable to get aid from the federal government and had to beg. The columnist took sympathy on this alleged vet, telling his horrible war and post-war story. I read the story and, if I didn't know better, would have also taken pity on this man. Instead, I called a health care reporter at the Free Press I knew. I told her the real story. She contacted the columnist and the story ended. Danny sure knew how to ride every opportunity to come his way. I don't know what happened to him. I never saw him again after that I day I saw him, nude, walking on his hands. Poor Danny.

Grant

He was a drinking alcoholic; an actively drinking alcoholic. In the three years we had a computer for patient registration, Grant managed fifty-six ED visits for a variety of minor medical problems-leg abrasions, colds, etc.—and one major—alcohol abuse Each time he came in, his blood alcohol was measured; I am not sure why we kept repeating it. Grant was always clinically drunk. His blood level never went down as far as 100; many times he made it close to 500. But he never was so drunk that he required intubation, like others. Sometimes he came in to get something to eat. Sometimes he came in to get out of the weather. Sometimes he just came in.

Loud to a fault, Grant usually bellowed from the entry to exit. He didn't, however; swear at the staff, nursing or medical. Usually his complaints had to do with pain in his left leg, where he had an abrasion for as long as I can remember. Sometimes he complained of pain in his arm. Nothing was ever found of any medical significance. Clean shaven at times, when I saw him last, he had a full beard and thick, bushy hair. He was getting gray.

Grant had health insurance, not the best but not the worst. But he continued to come to us, never to his primary care physician. I am not sure what his total bills were, but I am sure that they were significant. He never had any cash and often slept on the street. Every attempt made to refer him to an alcohol rehabilitation center, failed; he just refused to go. I am not sure that even today he considers his alcohol abuse a problem. The rumor was that he had a wife, but I never saw her. There finally came a time when he would be seen, no chart made out and he was removed.

Betsy

Betsy was a middle aged woman. She had sustained a closed head injury in an auto accident, following which she had seizures. Sometimes she even took her medicine; but usually not. And when she did, she washed them down with alcohol. Most of her nutrition was in the form of liquids—usually, alcohol.

Betsy made her money selling her body, such as it was. Actually, she leased it out. She sustained another auto accident, which produced some internal injuries requiring a colostomy. When she was discharged, she again became financially independent by returning to a self-employed state. A frequent flyer, most often it was because she had a seizure. But there were other things that brought her in, including infection. While in the hospital, for completeness sake, a house officer took a swab of her colostomy. It grew out gonorrhea. Betsy brought new meaning to the phrase, "making money on the side."

Joan

One night, I was working in the treatment rooms, mostly in Module 3, at DRH. There was a middle aged woman-Joan- with a split lower lip. She was a mean drunk and had put on her hospital gown so it was open in front. She didn't tie it closed, just held it.

I approached Joan in my best bedside manner. Introduced myself and asked what the problem was. She told me she had been hit in the face and her lip split open. Joan was an angry drunk that night.

I put on gloves and reached for lip. "Don't touch my lip."

"I have to see if you need stitches or your teeth have been knocked loose."

"Don't touch my fucking lip." I reached for it and touched it. She went bananas. "You mother fucker. I told you not to touch my lip!" She was off the gurney in a flash, charging me. I backed away as fast as I could. She kept coming at me while I ran in the other direction, into the main ED. I turned to see her coming, her large sagging breasts flapping in the breeze; her gown open. She was nude under the gown. I kept running; she kept screaming. I was laughing; staff was laughing, as I ran in and out of the other modules. Finally two nursing staff, still laughing, restrained her and put her on a gurney. Someone else sewed her up.

Archie

Archie, not his real name, was an elderly man who, I think, started to come after we opened at DRH. He was an older man, who hobbled in, with his cane, periodically. Actually his visits became more and more frequent as time went on. Archie always wore multiple layers of clothing, even in the summer. His visits were always on the afternoon shift. His complaint was also always the same: constipation. Initially, he received, against his own desires, a complete evaluation to insure he did not have cancer, or any other cause of mechanical bowel obstruction. When the evaluation indicated no cause, he was treated with stool softeners, and sent home. But this wasn't good enough for Archie.

When he left us, he walked almost two miles to our sister hospital, Hutzel, where he was seen again, since all ED's had a moral and ethical, perhaps legal, obligation to see and treat all comers. There he was evaluated, given a bottle of citrate of magnesia and sent home.

The next day, the very next day, he repeated the cycle. This time, however, he insisted, and got, another bottle of citrate of magnesia. This kept going on until he died. Sometimes he modified his circular pattern and went first to Hutzel. Archie never had any other complaint besides constipation. Sometimes to avoid an early repeat visit he was given two bottles of citrate, which he took at the same time.

There were times when he came in covered with feces because he could no longer exert bowel control. He would be cleaned up and discharged, to once again restart his cycle. In time, he became more and more cantankerous; and our staff became less and less tolerant, no longer seeing it as a joke. He was treated with more hostility and he became more hostile. Archie began swinging his cane at people, and became more demanding. Finally, one day he mouthed off to one of our attendings, and swung his cane. The attending responded in kind, and struck Archie. It was reported to me and I spoke to the involved doc, who told me he had just snapped. The doc was disciplined by me. But the hospital administration wanted more and his hospital privileges were suspended for a time.

Archie in Room 3; really sick.
Entry: 7/20/81
Floater: Krome
Archie birthday Friday
Entry: 3/15/82
Floater: JET

Then Archie died. In the hospital.

Stella

DGH was located just at one edge of Greek Town; a center of action even today; multiple Greek restaurants, bakeries, bars, and today a casino. Stella was a Greektown fixture, wandering the streets, dressed in a white nurse's uniform (I don't know where she got it), and

98

an Eisenhower jacket with sergeant's stripes. She was schizophrenic, but harmless. Stella would go store to store selling little bags of peanuts. I still don't know where she got them or the jacket. She took no medications of which I am aware. Walking the streets, she would stop and talk to the voices only she could hear, sometimes loudly. No one mugged her or struck her. The Greentown people would say hello and keep walking; the police knew her

Every winter, when it started to get cold, and snowy, the police brought her in to the psychiatrists. She would be committed to NSH (Northville State Hospital) until spring. Then the cycle would begin again. I don't know what happened to her, but she lives in the memory of those of us who worked at DGH.

The Vibrator Incident

One evening, I'm not sure when, B. was working in Room 6, the male medical room, when a homosexual sat down beside him.

Dr. B: What's the problem, tonight?
Patient: I am gay.
Dr. B.: And......
Patient: I have a vibrator in my rectum.
Long silence.
Dr. B.: Well, we can do one of three things.
Patient: What?
Dr. B.: We can turn it off. We can remove it. Or we replace the batteries. Your choice.
It was removed. True story.

The Two Tampon Lady

I was working days in ARC (Ambulatory Reception Center). It was in the middle of my shift and I grabbed the next chart. I read the

Triage note. *"Sent from health department clinic because she has a tampon stuck in her vagina"*; not an unusual complaint, but not a common one.

The patient told me she had two tampons stuck in her vagina. The doctors at the clinic, according to the patient, couldn't get them out. So she was sent to us. And I was the lucky doctor the fates assigned to the task. I went through three plastic vaginal speculums and two ring forceps and finally had to use my hand to get all the pieces out. A student nurse was assisting me and I am sure she will remember this for all time. It took forty minutes to remove all the fragments. In that interval, ten more patients arrived.

The Taxi and the Psych Patient

One evening, I am not sure of the time or date, but the incident was in the Log, a woman who was in the Crisis Center was discharged. She refused to go and was angry and yelling. She had no choice and a cab had been ordered to take her home. In an attempt to convince everybody of how crazy she was, she went into the ladies room and came out stark naked. It didn't work. Everyone told her to put her clothes on and get in the cab. The cab had arrived and the driver was in the lobby waiting for her.

When she realized that, she got dressed in one of the treatment rooms, walked out the ambulance entrance, down the ramp, and stole the cab. I am not sure the driver ever got it back.

Through the Front Door

One night we discharged, ejected, an angry drunk. He was furious about the treatment he had received and about being ejected. He walked down the ambulance ramp to the street, where he got into his car, and gunned it, drove up the ramp to the front door, and drove right into the lobby through the door.

Andrew

I couldn't decide whether to put Andrew in this section or in "Our Bad." He was a patient who, in fact, we made bad. He was a young, black man, with sickle cell disease who was a regular to the DMC hospitals. Andrew is an example of many of the "sicklers," as we called them. All who came in with sickle cell pain crisis were treated with re-hydration, either IV or by mouth, and narcotics for pain. Andrew made getting legal narcotics an art form.

Often when he first started to come in with pain, he had a complete evaluation. No medical cause was ever found. Not until 2004 when he died at another hospital. I guess this time he was really sick. The drill with Andrew changed over time, but he most often got a narcotic—Dilaudid, and Benadryl. And he had to get two doses of each before he said he was pain free. Often in one day Andrew would visit us twice; once in the morning and once in the evening.

Between visits to us, Andrew would visit Harper and Hutzel, with the same pitch. We only knew about those when we had the computer network up. He had favorite doctors and would call in and ask who was on duty. When he found out someone was on who didn't treat him the way he wanted, Andrew would by-pass DRH and go to another hospital.

Andrew was hospitalized several times at DRH and Harper over the years. He had insurance, Medicare, and even had a hematologist as a private physician. But this didn't break the cycle. It reached the point that EMS refused to pick him up; so he would contact a private ambulance service. Andrew was even arrested once for forging prescriptions. The police brought him to DRH.

But we created the substance abuse problem for Andrew and other sicklers. Oral medications didn't work. Prescriptions never lasted; so we gave narcotics. I don't mean to imply that all the sicklers were drug seekers. Oh, there were some; but not all. Some kept their clinic appointments and only came in rarely. Andrew and several others had the substance personalities, and we feed into them.

I just called DRH to get some information about Andrew and was told he had died at Sinai Hospital in November 2004. I couldn't believe it. I always thought he was immortal.

The Old Lady and God

Lots of our patients had deep religious beliefs and superstitions. We had to learn to deal with their beliefs and get the patient to the point of accepting medical help. Many believed that their health was in God's hands. Once when a patient said they had to pray on what to do, B. went into the cubicle, and said he would pray with them.

Chapter XIV
Busy Day

"Very busy day
3 critical GSW
2 cardiac arrests
————-at noon in ED; handled without a hitch"
Entry 3/3/76
Floater: T.

Five critical patients in one hour were unusual; but it happened. There could be as many as three critical cases in a shift and as few as one a day. When the sun went down, things picked up and there might be as many as five cases going in the OR at the same time. Although most of the patients had been stabbed, in the mid seventies the number of gunshot wounds began to exceed the number of stab wounds.

There were the usual automobile accidents, pedestrian accidents and motorcycle accidents. People continued to fall off roof tops and ladders. In the winter, there were house fires, with the attendant smoke inhalation victims as well as burns; in the summer, patients walked on hot charcoal, not in a religious fervor, but inadvertently. Interpersonal trauma always increased in the summer. Our busiest month was always August; the hottest month.

Always there was the continuous undercurrent of non-trauma cases: cardiac patients, pneumonia, hypertension, alcohol and drug abuse, suicides, etc.

Sometime in the early '80s a sixteen-year-old boy was in a motorcycle accident that left him a quadriplegic. The motorcycle was a birthday gift from his father just that day. The father was completely torn up, crying, and sobbing, sitting on a stool next to his son holding his hand; a truly sad scene. Ironically, my second son had been pushing me to buy him a motorcycle for his sixteenth birthday. Today he was doing semi-volunteer work in the ED; semi because if he didn't have a real job, that paid, he had to work as a volunteer at the hospital. So did his brother.

I brought my son over, hoping this would convince him and offer justification for my denial. We stood where we could see the patient lying on a gurney, IV's running and a neck collar in place. I told my son the patient's story. He looked me in the eye and said, "He just didn't know what he was doing, Dad."

I gave up. "You are not getting a motorcycle as long as you live at home. When you move out you can make up your own mind."

Hospital closed last night physician staff couldn't handle the load

6 critical cases on board code going –another in status epilepticus

Entry: 3/11/80

Floater: JMN

Another typical day.

We were being sued for the wrongful death of a young girl with a ruptured atrium, a lethal injury; four of us, the hospital and the sending hospital and the EMT's who took her to, what turned out to be, the sending hospital. I don't remember the outcome, but I hadn't thought we committed malpractice, and none of the docs paid. When any patient died, it never was because of the disease, it was always because of the doctor, the nurse, or the hospital. Oh, there was plenty of malpractice. The single biggest cause of malpractice was malpractice.

Malpractice premiums always went up. I graduated med school in 1961, and it seems to me that every twenty years or so, we had a malpractice crisis, when we couldn't get insurance, or the premiums were so high we couldn't afford it. When I started my training I had to buy my own insurance. It was no big deal: thirty-five dollars for coverage up to one to two hundred thousand.

Malpractice insurance coverage was a major issue for the ED medical staff. I had been told that there was a city ordinance that covered us. Wrong. The ordinance was supposed to cover city employees and "special others." In addition many of us provided services for community functions and we were unsure if the ordinance would, or did, cover us. For example, our activities at rock concerts, covering automobile races, acting as medical resource for Detroit EMS and giving radio orders to the paramedics, providing medical care at free clinics. We needed something in writing to insure our coverage. The hospital administrator wrote the city law office for clarification.

Being a good city bureaucracy, the reply was a long time coming. If we had to buy our own, assuming we could, it was really going to cost a lot, really a lot. I got estimates and passed them on to the hospital administrator. The whole thing was reaching crisis proportions; crisis creation was the way we often got things done working with the city.

So it was my turn to create a crisis. I sent a memo to the hospital administrator complaining about the whole thing. He sent one back, telling me in essence, he didn't understand what I had written. I put a hand written note on the bottom of his memo and sent it back. "Fuck you, strong note to follow." Then I sent a strong note (I liked sending memos!).

I outlined, again, the problem, and told him if we didn't have it straight in two weeks, all of the emergency medical staff would leave! One of my full timers leaked the memo to a reporter for the Detroit Free Press. I, of course, went out of town to a meeting. In two weeks we had a letter informing me and all the others of our coverage, which included any work approved by me. Another crisis; another resolution!

I have been, until today, named in about ten suits. Mostly it because I was chief and had to have policies in place to protect patients, and taken steps to make sure the policies were followed.

But I was named in suits where I was a treating doctor. In August 1969, I was served with papers naming me in a suit for the first time. I just finished my residency in July. After I read the papers, I immediately called my insurance agent, who told me not to read them. Too late. "Well, don't take it personally."

"First of all, mine is the name on here, not yours. Second, he doesn't have anything nice to say about me. In fact, he says some very nasty things. Finally, I am being sued for $250,000 when I only have about $450 dollars in the bank." I knew I didn't do anything wrong; the patient was managed in a textbook fashion. Everything done was clearly indicated. I had a pre-op note that said she understood and I had explained what was likely to be done.

Basically, this was an eighteen-year-old lady seen in consultation when I was a senior surgery resident. She had been laparoscoped by the gynecologist as part of an infertility work-up. I was called to see her some six weeks after she had been discharged and returned to be hospitalized for abdominal pain. I suspected an abdominal abscess. My attending and I explored her and found peritoneal pus and a perforated sigmoid diverticulum. A diverting colostomy was done. She had a hectic course, including three days in the ICU. Subsequently, she was discharged and was re-admitted six weeks later and had the colostomy repaired. Her post-operative course was without further complication. I remember the young lady very well. Because of her, I was no longer a malpractice virgin. You always remember your first.

But I was scared. No, I was terrified. I called the agent who handled my house insurance and asked that my personal liability be increased to one million dollars. He called back to tell me my insurance couldn't be raised because I was already involved in a liability suit. Shit.

Nine months later, I went to the plaintiff lawyer's office to give a deposition. When I came in with my lawyer, the plaintiff attorney told me his client was dropping the suit. "Forgive us Dr. Krome, sometimes these things are started before we have all the facts."

"Funny, when I do that you call it malpractice." The suit went away. The gynecologist counter sued and won.

I was also named in a suit, the details of which I don't remember except I was accused of bigotry, and, therefore, biased against her client. I and the hospital both won that one.

A patient was transferred from another hospital because of a lack of insurance. He had been there about six hours. I was in the ER, taking call for the trauma service. The resident called me to see the patient who had a gunshot of the right groin. There were no pulses distal from the gunshot wound. The patient couldn't move his foot at the ankle. Sensation was also absent. We boarded him to repair a gunshot wound involving the femoral artery. I told the patient that I felt that his leg was severely injured and he might well lose his lower leg. He understood and signed the surgical consent form. I made a complete pre-op note. Two years later the patient lost his foot. He sued me, and several others. I was dropped because of my pre-op note.

Talk about busy days. On July 12, 1969, a thirty-nine-foot cabin cruiser exploded on the Detroit River, at a marina, near Belle Isle. Twenty people were on board, including eight kids under thirteen. Nineteen were transferred to the hospital; one to a close by hospital; eighteen to us. Two were DOA, two died later. All burned kids were on gurneys watching the events in the ER. Fourteen in all were hospitalized. All the patients had to have their burns washed, dressed; IV's started and medication given. The critical cases were intubated. Within an hour of arrival, all were treated and either discharged or hospitalized. Families were contacted, news releases issued. The incident was over. It was the first disaster on my watch. Police and firefighters had brought all the patients quickly and efficiently. The ER personnel had functioned with a high level of professionalism.

Chapter XV
Helicopter

Like most wars, the Vietnam War had a significant impact on civilian medical care, mostly emergency medicine and surgery. There was a new respect for the concept that trauma patients belonged in trauma centers as early as possible. Movement of the injured to centers as expeditiously as possible was part and parcel of their care and that movement was enhanced by the helicopter. After the war, both pilots and helicopters were returned to the US. Surplus helicopters were released to public service agencies, and pilots returned looking for work.

EMS providers and law enforcement agencies throughout the US became interested in the use of helicopters. There was a need for rapid transport to major trauma centers; and, as evidence showed in Vietnam, there was a medical advantage for patients if they could be moved directly to trauma centers from the scene.

There was an advantage for hospitals who ran helicopter services; economics. It was costly to operate a helicopter service. But the financial return was great because the service brought in new patients from beyond the usual hospital service area. In addition, a significant number of these required the operating room and an intensive care unit bed. Each trauma patient brought in spent six to ten days in an ICU. Lots of money for the hospital.

Because not all areas of Michigan had access to trauma centers, helicopter services allowed patients living in rural areas to gain access in a reasonable time. Pediatric patients could be transferred to children's hospitals. There were, of course, patients who required sophisticated cardiac care and they could be flown to the medical center as well. Finally, a trauma team could be brought to the scene, to begin care.

In Detroit, the helicopter service began as a cooperative effort between DRH and the Aviation Division of the DPD (Detroit Police Department). In the mid-'70s, pilots from the division of aviation approached us to determine our level of interest in starting a medical evacuation service. We had no helipad, but the police assured us they could land in a vacant lot across the street from the hospital, between two apartment towers. The helicopter would remain based at Detroit City Airport, where the service was housed. A call would be received by the floater requesting the transport. Aviation would determine availability of the helicopter (weather, etc.). As time progressed, the floater would be called with notification of availability before we even got a request. The pilots would determine the availability of the copter; the floater, medical necessity.

DPD acquired two Huey helicopter gun ships, stripped of all guns and armament. One was put to use, the other was kept for parts. A number of pilots were hired by the city, but not with the idea of running a medical service. Some of the pilots, however, had flown Medivac airships in 'Nam. One pilot had actually flown the Huey we obtained.

So, we had a Huey for transfers, one for parts, four pilots experienced with the Hueys, and a plan. We trained the pilots to the level of EMT's. The ER would provide the training through our existing training programs. Medical supplies were provided by DRH and Children's Hospital (CHM). If the transfer was a neonate (newborn) or infant, CHM provided the staff, incubator and ventilation equipment. We provided a doctor and nurse or two doctors to fly.

Across the nation, there was a rapid growth in the number of services. There were five serving southeast Michigan alone. Sometimes when we were flying we would see another in the air. Not all the flying around was safe; one year there were five crashes with deaths of pilots, paramedics, doctors, and, of course, nurses.

Flying in the copter was voluntary. When we had residents, flying was optional for them as well. Usually, one of the more senior emergency physicians went on the flight. Although I didn't like flying at all, I flew too.

The call would come in to the floater, who verified availability, if it wasn't already done. He would notify aviation we had a flight. Sometimes we drove out to city airport; usually we drove to the landing site. If the transfer was to a Medical Center hospital, security would arrange for an ambulance or EMS to meet us and off board the patient. When the patient was critical we would land in the street in front of the hospital.

The service operated until about one year after we moved into DRH. Despite our requests and suggestions, no helipad was built close to the hospital. We used a helipad about a quarter of mile away. But it wasn't satisfactory. Then, some administrators in the aviation service got in trouble and retired or resigned. It didn't affect our pilots. But it was enough to put a nail in the coffin.

We enjoyed the service and it was valuable. In the beginning, we made a number of public relations flights, demonstrating the helicopter and lecturing on preparing a patient. The number of transfers to DMC (Detroit Medical Center) hospitals began to increase, mostly for CHM (Children's Hospital of Michigan). We were bringing in three to five new patients daily for the DMC; the cost was more than the revenue generated. It was, however, good public relations.

After we off boarded the patient, the pilots would take us flying. Sometimes we would fly over Tiger stadium, hover, watch a little of the game and catch the scores on the scoreboard. One time, after paramedics, firefighters and police had been trained in high-rise rescue and rappelling, we put on a demonstration on Police Day at the stadium. The pilots offered me the opportunity to rappel with them. I declined, but did watch.

When we had to return to the apartment vacant lot, the pilots would hover in landing, and we would look in to the windows and check things out!

When we flew, all of us kept our eyes pealed looking for wires, radio towers, etc. Medical equipment was placed in the helicopter, and we sat on a portable gurney wearing head phones and microphones to communicate with the pilot and co-pilot. In front of us was the medical equipment. We prepared what we needed as we flew. The medical staff didn't have helmets, and the seat belts were used to fix the gurney so it didn't roll around. I tell you all this for a specific reason.

We were returning to the airport. There were two doctors on board; me and JET. The pilot turned to us and said, "Put on your helmets."

"We don't have helmets."

"Put on your seatbelts."

"We don't have seatbelts." Things weren't looking good. "What's going on, Rick."

"Nothing terrible. We lost hydraulics. We'll have to land like an airplane. Hold on." We held on for dear life, but nothing happened.

It was snowing, hard. Not unusual for Detroit. We got a call for Medivac. The pilots said we could fly. It looked like a blizzard to me. I talked to our chief pilot. No problem. But the expressways were unusable because of the snow. There was no way I could get to the landing site, or the airport. They had already picked up a nurse. They were willing to come to my house, using the helicopter, to pick me up; if there was someplace they could land. There was an elementary school right across the street. It being night, there were no lights. They called Southfield police who secured the field, surrounded it with police cars with turned on head lights.

My daughter has cerebral palsy. She was watching from our front room, standing on the bed. When the helicopter came in she got so excited, she began bouncing on the bed. I think she even wet herself.

One day, we received a call from EMS that they needed a doctor at the scene. We dispatched the helicopter, with two doctors and one nurse on board. EMS felt that the patient, whose leg was trapped in a piece of heavy equipment, might require an amputation. I got an amputation knife, while the nurse and the other doctor assembled the IV's and sedation, just in case. The flight was about five minutes, and we landed in small lot just outside the plant. All three of us walked into the plant on wooden planks. The planks were over what looked like

111

sludge and smelled like feces. I commented to one of workers, who told the nurse that this was a solid waste processing plant.

Great! I made up my mind not to do an amputation in the midst of all this shit. The trapped worker's leg was in the middle of a piece of heavy equipment, wrapped around a large gear. There was no way to get him out without the amputation, which I was sure would kill him. We started an IV. I asked the workers to be prepared to lift the gear and pull him out. We shot him up with IV narcotics and sedation. When he fell asleep, I gave the word. He was extracted and placed on a gurney, flown to DRH, taken to the OR; his leg amputated, but he survived. If he felt pain, he never showed it.

Medivac transfer yesterday. One hundred percent burn child with facial and nasal burns not intubated.

Transferred to CHM.
Entry: 9/14/77
Floater: BCW

This is where the helicopter paid off. Especially for kids.

Good Medivac flight by Dr. S. last PM with 80% burn victim.
Admitted here.
Entry: 9/23/77
Floater: BCW
2 Medivac flights yesterday includes 1 nite flight (first one)
Entry: 11/3/77
Floater: JMN

The number of flights was increasing. Multiple flights daily were becoming more common. It was too bad that we were not destined to have a helipad at DRH. The chairman of the board decided it was more important to have a lithotripsy machine than a helicopter service. In typical fashion I wasn't asked and couldn't present any data to support the financial impact of the helicopter service.

Chapter XVI
Residents and Nurses

John Doe #81 was seen by surgery as possible GI bleeder (bleeding from the gastrointestinal tract). Patient released by surgery but not dispositioned (discharged or admitted) –amylase 350; alcohol 300. Will repeat bloods—meantime patient had another seizure.
Entry: 04/76
Floater: JMN

A clear hospitalization! Another example of your unsupervised residents in action. Or rather lack of action.

Surgical residents gave us problems over the years. It was as though they still felt that the ER was their domain to run as they sought fit. They frequently held patients over night because they didn't want the patients admitted to wards they didn't like. And their rapport with the nursing staff, in general, left something to be desired. On top of that, they didn't have much respect for our medical staff. I can't say that I blamed them. Our staff was mostly moonlighters and what full timers we had didn't know as much as the senior surgical residents.

Unsupervised residents in all specialties were a problem in the '60s through the early '80s. Consulting residents would see patients, and make whatever disposition they thought was appropriate. If they represented a surgical service, and the patient was to be hospitalized or scheduled for an operation, the attending was called. If the patient was discharged, it was without any further discussion. Patients who were admitted were seen by the attending within twelve hours. No one went for an operation unless seen by the attending surgeon first. If a patient was hospitalized erroneously, they wound up spending a needless night in the hospital. If he was sent home erroneously, well, then he could get in trouble. I was most concerned about those sent home who should have stayed.

On some wards the care at night left a great deal to be desired. Because I had trained here, I was acutely aware of this problem. So at night some patients were kept until morning in the emergency room, and I couldn't fault the residents even though it contributed to the crowding.

The demand for trained emergency physicians far and away exceeded the supply. Residencies in emergency medicine didn't get started until 1971 and we didn't start ours until 1976. The environment was difficult to say the least. Not many, if any, academic institutes wanted to get involved in the education and training of students and residents in emergency medicine. We needed, and a lot of other hospitals did too, enough full time, trained emergency physicians to make our presence felt around the clock. We had to cut out moonlighters. There is little doubt in my mind we couldn't have made it through these trying times without them. They didn't attend staff meetings, were unaware of policies or policy changes, and had little respect from the nurses or other medical staff.

In the 1980s, I left and a new chief was brought in and the pieces started to fall into place. Nothing succeeds like a successor.

Disciplining residents for major offenses was never a major problem; for minor problems, it was virtually an everyday occurrence. Most of the residents were committed to medicine, and their own specialty training. Every once in a while, just every once in a while, one over stepped the bounds of ethical and moral limits.

One evening I was working in my office at DRH, when two

security officers came to my door. "Dr. Krome, there is a big problem. According to a woman, one of your doctors took her to an eighth floor on-call room and fondled her. She can and has identified him."

"Whoa, we don't even have an eighth floor, and there are no on-call rooms. But I'll talk to him."

I called the resident in off the floor. He, of course denied everything. I sent him back to work, taking him at face value. The security people brought in the complainant's statement. It was very detailed, telling us which elevator had been used and where she was taken. It made sense and sounded true. I brought the resident back in and confronted him with the statement. He now admitted he had taken her upstairs, but denied fondling her.

There was nothing I could do but suspend him from the emergency department for the remainder of his month. I called his residency director, told him what had happened, and forwarded all statements to him. I also told him the involved resident was not to come back to the emergency department, not even as a consultant. The program director could do what he wanted; I was going to notify administration. I never saw the resident and heard he was placed on probation for a year.

There appears to be rebellion of the RN staff protesting the appointment of LB, RN as head nurse.

Four nurses had called in sick; a not unusual incident when they wanted to protest; at times we didn't even know what the protest was about! One showed up for work, saw how many had come in and immediately signed out. Of the four who had called in, two were supervisors. An interesting mess, made worse by the complicity of the shift supervisors. The RN's, LPN's, and nursing supervisors all had separate unions. When one went out, the others usually went out too, in a show of union solidarity.

Improving the nursing, both levels of staffing and quality, was a top priority. To enrich their jobs, and give them a better sense of self esteem, we needed lots of changes. The director of nursing, someone

I came to respect and even admire, in later years was against my making changes. She perceived, and rightly so, that these changes might instill in all nurses a search for job enhancement and a sense of self-assertiveness that would come down to her losing control of the nursing staff. In addition, there was no doubt nurses would ask for pay increases. There had to be a step by step logical progression of change.

When I started, RN's were not allowed to start IV's with medication in them, or add medications to already running IV's; they couldn't hang blood for transfusion, pass nasogastric tubes, or even apply certain dressings. They couldn't pass Foley catheters in opposite sex patients. Mostly what they did was keep the area clean and stocked; a lot of money for this level of education. There were nurses who bent the rules, sometimes to the point of breaking them. It was hard not to support them.

There was no continuing education program, and none were members of the Emergency Department Nursing Association, their professional organization. All wore the same uniform: white skirt, white blouse, and white nursing cap. Styles were changing and the nurses wanted a uniform change.

The first thing to go was the white caps. Traditional nurses felt that patients wouldn't be able to tell who they were without caps. The skirts were changed to pants, and in the summer, Bermuda shorts were allowed. Since some nurses didn't like them ("they'll make me look like a house") the changes were made optional.

With the support of the Head Nurse, and few of the others, a series of educational programs was begun, slowly upgrading performance and enhancing jobs. There were conflicts with the Director of Nursing who thought we were asking the nurses to work harder, and many of whom saw us teaching skills not generally required by the house nurses. Many, resistant to the changes, thought they were being asked to do things done by the residents and interns, making their jobs easier, and this was our primary motivation.

We needed a nurse to conduct the educational programs, do bedside teaching and organize nursing performance audits. Although the doctors did give some of the lectures; most were given by the nurses themselves.

To select an "in service educator," a note was sent to all registered nurses encouraging interested nurses to apply. From this pool the head nurse and I selected one with significant educational experience, who already taught at a community college. She was promoted to head nurse, with the clear understanding that she still had to work every other weekend and pull floor shifts. She was not a frontline supervisor.

The appointment, with promotion, of a white woman to what was considered a cushiony job, provoked a lot of anger from the other nurses; hence, today's sick calls.

We became a closed unit (nurses could not go out to the floors when they were short staffed, and we couldn't get help when we were short staff). New nurses had to have at least six months experience working in-house. When a new graduate nurse applied for a job, she was referred to the Nursing Director for possible employment before she could come down into the ER. Audits were started by nurses of charts to make sure that was being done for and to the patients was appropriate, recorded and followed existing policies. Nursing staff meetings for each shift were begun to discuss policy and policy changes; to review the results of nursing audits; and to listen to the nurses' complaints and suggestions. Criteria for the audits were developed by the nurses at their staff meetings. Educational programs included skills necessary for nurses to perform.

Nurses had to demonstrate these skills to continue to be employed in the ER. Each RN was given two years to successfully complete an ACLS course (Advanced Cardiac Life Support Course). Failure to complete one would result in her being moved out of the ER. All either successfully completed a course, or resigned before it even came up. In fact, most nurses got their certification and began teaching. It was a significant accomplishment and they took a lot of personal pride in it.

One of our fulltime physicians was course director for ACLS courses, which were expanded to include medical students, residents, and moonlighters; the moonlighters couldn't work in the ER until they successfully completed a course. The nurse educator became the second-in-command for these programs. Some of the residents objected to being taught by nurses; they got over it.

Morale was improving. Nursing staff numbers were increasing. The national shortage of nurses impacted us. I cannot remember a time, even when I retired, when we had a full complement of nurses.

Nowhere else in healthcare do nurses and physicians work as closely as they do in the ED. Nowhere else is the need as acute for well trained, educated and compassionate nursing staff as in the ED. Caring concerned nurses do more for the patients, visitors, and doctors than anyone else.

They flew on our helicopters as volunteers; no extra pay. They worked long hours under brutal conditions in each of the disasters and riots that occurred in Detroit. They taught in our educational programs. They were part of our evaluation system of doctors and residents. They went to public schools to teach. They conducted education programs in churches and in the community. They were there when Detroit had the auto races as volunteers, and camped on Belle Isle when the Boy Scouts had their Jamboree.

During my internship, the police brought in an unconscious woman, breathing on her own, but not responsive to painful stimuli. She moaned, occasionally. I checked her pupils, blood pressure and pulse. Nothing unusual. I was barely one month out of medical school. No clue about what was happening. I put an airway in her mouth; she didn't gag. I started an IV with 5% dextrose/water, the standard solution of the day. As I leaned back to survey the situation, a registered nurse, not a young one, slid a syringe with a needle on it into my hand. *"Here is what you asked for Doctor."* I hadn't asked for anything. I gave the medicine, not knowing what it was, but relying on the nurse's judgment, intravenously. Almost before I could get the syringe out, the patient woke up and began talking clearly. To me it was a miracle; to the nurse, hypoglycemia in a diabetic. I have relied on nurses' judgments ever since.

To expedite patient movement, and operate more efficiently, the triage system was modified to use experienced nursing staff as triage officers. A full time emergency physician was put in charge and was responsible for monitoring the system, including the performance of the triage nurses. He also had regular meetings and special education programs for them. In what would later be called advanced triage, the nurses were allowed, after appropriate training, to order extremity x-rays and urinalysis.

Patients could be triaged to: (one) "Screening," the area designed for patients who had minor injuries or medical problems; (two) the acute treatment areas, based on their sex, and if there was trauma involved; (three) the psych crisis center. Patients mistakenly triaged to an acute treatment area could not be re-triaged to screening; patients triaged to screening could be re-triaged to an acute treatment area.

The system worked well, and, though modified, is still in existence. Originally designed to handle walk-in patients, it has been expanded to include EMS patients. Many patients had called 911 to get an ambulance to come to the hospital because they didn't have a ride and couldn't afford a taxi. At triage they were converted to walking status and triaged to Screening. The premise for the staff selected, was they had to be the most experienced. They were. Whenever, for training purposes, a resident, medical student, or EMT student was allowed to be in triage, the system would falter.

In 1980, one of our first triage nurses, a fine woman, committed to our ED, hard working and diligent, was operated on for a brain tumor. I really liked her, as did most others. She had a unique ability to relate to our patients and knew most of our groupys on a first name basis. She was pleasant, soft spoken, generally, and she made fantastic corn bread, which she periodically brought in for departmental parties. She came back to work after surgery, wearing a wig. But she wasn't the same. I can still see her in my mind's eye. She and another LPN was the core of our triage team. I miss them both.

There were two older nurses who came with the ER when I started. These nurses started the shift by ignoring patients and cleaning up the treatment area. They both went on to retire or return to the city when the new hospital started. But one filed a union grievance when someone else got promoted. Although she was black and the appointed head nurse was white she did not claim racial discrimination. What she did claim was the selection process was unfair because it was not based on seniority. This was a union shop and most if not all promotions were based on seniority. She lost her grievance; it was a landmark case for the hospital.

Chapter XVII
Ejected

*Psych brought up problem of psych pt. MC #173410, 4/9/76.
Pt. was discharged; refused to go-got violent. Psych approached
guards who then refused to eject pt. saying they had no authority
to deal with mental patients. This appears clear cut. (a) if pt. has
not been discharged the doctors can treat pt as necessary; (b) if
pt. has been discharged, then this becomes a civil case and the
route should be through civil authorities, administration and
their guards. The hooker is that it never looks good when an
attempt to eject a patient is started.*
Entry: 4/12/76
Floater: JNM

Although this case involved a psychiatric patient, it also occurred
with non-psych patients. Patients who felt that their treatment was
inadequate for any reason sometimes refused to leave. Some were
mad at their doctors, nurses, or other staff. Some lost control,
threatening the staff and otherwise acting out. In these instances, it
was sometimes necessary to step in; try to calm everyone down; and
eventually, at times, remove the patient or the visitors. They could be
arrested for trespassing; some were.

At DGH, the security officers left a great deal to be desired. They were unarmed (thank God), and didn't carry anything that could even be construed as a weapon. I don't know why they were even hired.

No one really wanted to eject a patient or visitor. No one was sure how much jeopardy they would be in, or if, administration would back them up if the fan went off. If it made the papers, security and the rest of staff would feel the heat. And the heat could come from hospital administration or from the city fathers, or both. I certainly understood why everyone was reluctant to get involved in this stuff. But it had to be done. When it hit the headlines, it would read, *"Sick man refused treatment at DRH," "Patient kicked out of DRH."* Not good publicity.

Very warm day. Engineering still hasn't taken care of air conditioner for Emergency Department.
Entry: 4/16/76
Floater: JMN

What we called "engineering" was in reality maintenance, construction and engineering. They were responsible for repair and relatively minor construction and would arrange for the city's construction team to come in.

I have already described the emergency department, but not the changes made by our first pass at reconstruction. The first room on the right on entry from the ambulance was converted to a single patient shock room, with operating room lights and cabinets in stainless steel. It became, in effect, a resuscitation room for trauma and non-trauma patients.

The second, was converted to a trauma room with an attached suture room; both small and crowded. New cabinets were put in the trauma and suture rooms. And a new scrub sink. Ah, the scrub sink. The reconstruction occurred in the summer, with the last piece being the scrub sink. It was a hot week and we were coming up on a Friday night. We needed the sink for the weekend; I pushed hard on the supervisor, telling him everything had to be ready for sundown Friday.

As a last act, the sink was completed, and the supervisor took me in to see it. It looked fine and we opened the room for use.

After the first patient came in, the nurse called me to check out the sink. As I walked back with her, I told her I had already seen the sink. She didn't say anything just walked. When we got to the sink I stood back. *"Watch,* "she said. She turned on the water which drained all over the floor. She turned on the hot water; none, only cold. I felt so stupid. Buckets were placed under the drain pipes. They had to be emptied several times each shift. We used the room and the sink. To this day, I can't believe it! I never looked under the sink! The drain pipes had never been hooked up!

Another famous error by maintenance was the air conditioning. For years after the new air conditioning was installed at DGH, it would not functioning properly. The air conditioning would stop in the summer and turn on in the winter. We finally figured out that the thermostats were wired backwards; turning off in the summer and on in the winter; just the way they were set.

But I did learn how to read construction drawings; also that you can only trust two people, me and you. And I worry about you!

My ability to read construction drawings and blueprints paid off for me later, especially when we began building and planning for the new hospital. But even before that, I had a job offer in Arizona, at a hospital that was in the midst of planning for its reconstruction of the emergency room. It was, and is, a famous hospital, so I'll leave out its name. I went to visit. The interview went well and I was impressed. They showed me the blueprints for their new emergency room. Quickly, I saw that they had left out piped in oxygen lines. They never saw the error, until I pointed it out. I never took the job. The construction had little to do with my decision.

The chief of engineering was a nice man. I liked him, but had to watch him carefully when it came to construction or repairs. He wore a suit, tie, and white shirt everyday to work. He was a very natty dresser.

One time he came to my office with a medical problem. It was middle of the week. He had a headache and pain across the bridge of his nose. He was due to see his own doctor at the end of the week. He had been under treatment for sinus headaches, and needed something for the headache. There were no other neurological signs and he had no vision problems. I didn't do a complete physical, just talked to him. Two weeks later he was dead from a brain tumor. I don't know if his complaints were from the brain tumor, but I wouldn't be surprised if they were. I felt guilty as hell; still do; it seems to me I should have done something different. I don't know what. But I won't forget the incident.

Need revision of AMA (Against Medical Advise) procedure. Another 17 y/o signed out AMA while drunk
    Entry: 4/14/76
    Floater: JET

Having patients sign out AMA was not really tricky, but we managed to confuse the issue repeatedly. We didn't allow intoxicated or other impaired patients, to sign out. Nor could we allow psychiatrically disturbed patients to sign out, or minors; patients who had attempted suicide could not be signed out by family. But we had lots of patients who did go AMA. So we reviewed the policy for everyone and made it the physician's responsibility to get it signed and to make a note in the chart. The number fell.

Nearly everybody one hour late today due to DST (Daily Savings Time). Super Cool was only one on time.
    Entry: 4/24/76
    Floater: JET

Super cool was emergency medical technicians. I don't remember his real name. He was, however, unique. Hard working and diligent when at work, he would strut down the halls, wearing gold necklaces, gold bracelets, and lots of rings. He always wore shades. Everybody called him super cool. His absenteeism exceeded every one in the department. In fact, we once figured he was only at work twenty percent of the work week. But when he came, he couldn't be touched. Long hours and hard work. He was especially good establishing rapport with patients and visitors. He had a knack for minimizing confrontations.

I talked to him many times about his coming to work. He never changed. When we closed the old hospital, he didn't come with us.

Mr. Cool went home ill this AM "head hurts" 3 absences this week two absences last week no more paid sick time
Entry: 3/28/80
Floater: BCW
Why are the docs smoking in the rooms?

Entry: 4/24/76
Floater: T

These were the days when smoking was allowed. In the hospital there were no restricted areas. But we did make policy that one could not smoke in the treatment rooms or at patient bedside. The policy had to be made because doctors would make rounds and smoke. Regretfully, there were violators, myself included. I didn't smoke at bedside, but I did in the halls or at the nursing station or in my office. We had one faculty member who smoked a pipe, and he smoked everywhere. No one made an issue of it. When we moved to DRH, there was a desk for the docs to sit at and write, I smoked there and staff even put out an ashtray. When I was a junior surgery resident, we had a cigar smoking senior resident. He frequently had an unlit cigar in his mouth while he changed dressings.

Chapter XVIII
Emergency Medicine Residency

Our residency starts tomorrow. I hope all goes well.
Entry6/30/76
Floater: BFB

This comment, simple as it sounds, in truth, represented much work by many people. Just thanking those who shared the vision and helped would fill a book.

In July 1976, we began our own, our very own, residency in emergency medicine. And on July 1, two young men started and walked on the floor of the ED at significant professional peril. There was no approval mechanism for residency, no certifying board in emergency medicine, and no certifying examination in emergency medicine. These young men were betting their future careers on the development of all that by the time they finished their training in two years.

To begin a residency at a medical school first requires the creation of an academic unit. There are, basically, three options: (one) full academic department, (two) an academic program reporting directly to the dean; or, (three) a section of an existing academic department. The easiest is to create a section of an existing department; the

126

hardest, a full academic department. Since I was a member of the surgical faculty, the department of surgery seemed the best, and most logical, way to go. The department of surgery had to make emergency medicine a section of surgery. The chairman had been very supportive in the past. He had given up two fulltime faculty positions, which I divided into four positions. When, however, budget cuts occurred at the medical school, we lost one full time position; a decision made by the surgery chairman.

Our faculty taught in the medical school at the freshman, junior, and senior levels, with an introduction to emergency medical care for freshmen; juniors, with an ACLS course; and seniors, with a medical student elective in emergency medicine. One of our faculty was involved in basic (laboratory) research and had applied for, and obtained, grants. Others were doing clinical research and publishing. In essence, we were doing everything expected of an academic unit—-either a section or a department. We had more student contact hours than any other unit in the school. All of this in five to six short years. The only additional funds required would be to pay for the residents.

So, I met with the surgery chairman, armed with documentation of our academic accomplishments and a request he create a section of emergency medicine, which he could do with a stroke of the pen. He refused, saying emergency medicine wasn't a scientific discipline; didn't have enough research, etc., and it would be too expensive to create an academic unit.

This was a real roadblock. So the faculty met. We made two decisions. First, we would continue our commitment to education, research, the medical school, and to our patients. Second, we would go to the dean with a request that he do something. This would be going over the chairman's head. If he got pissed, he could, at the very least, cut off the financial benefit we currently enjoyed. I could find myself reassigned by him, and no longer have anything to do with emergency medicine.

The chairman of surgery, like all chairmen of academic departments, served at the pleasure of the dean, and was in fact, an officer of the school, and the dean had no intention of going around him.

We made a list of schools already in the business of starting, or running, residencies in emergency medicine. We wrote a curriculum, with objectives and goals for each rotation, in keeping with our definition of what the graduate should be able to do. BFB became our first residency program director. He sought input from our existing faculty and called directors of other residency programs at DRH. He developed a rotational schedule, and a list of objectives and goals for each rotation. The didactic schedule and the conferences were made by JET and became part of the educational programs for medical students. ACLS and ATLS programs were a part of the residency program.

My job was to find funding. I went to the hospital director, who said there was no money available to fund a new residency program. In fact, some residencies, not actively involved in providing health care at DGH, were going to take a cut. My homework, however; disclosed at least two departments, not taking hits, hadn't filed their programs in a number of years—medicine and surgery—and the rotating internship. He was open to our getting six positions——three for each of two years; if we could get the agreement of the chief of medicine and surgery. Each resident, in fact, required two years of funding; one for his junior year and one for his senior year. If we wanted the resident to start as an intern, then we would need an additional year of funding. An insurmountable task for surgery.

But he did agree to give us two positions from the internship pool. The others were my problem. The chief of medicine, after he realized he was going to get cut and also hadn't filled his residencies, agreed to give us two positions. I had to promise to return these positions if he should fill. Never happen. We were on our way. But that still left surgery to deal with.

I went back to the dean and gave him all the background on our funding, and the list, again, of all programs at medical schools. During the interval between our first and second meeting, I had gone to the Michigan Chapter of the American College of Emergency Physicians, many of whom were alumni. I told them we needed their help and asked that they start a letter writing campaign to the dean asking him to consider starting an academic unit so we could begin our residency. They did.

The dean began to understand we wouldn't go away. Evidently, he knew the chief of surgery wouldn't give up, so he did what all great deans do. He formed a committee. The membership consisted of three faculty, none from emergency medicine or surgery. The objective of the committee was to make a recommendation to the dean for the academic unit for emergency medicine. We knew we were home free and it was just a matter of time.

During this interval, and while I was negotiating, BFB and I began making the rounds of chiefs of those departments through which our residents would rotate. At each meeting, we presented our goals and objectives, listened to their comments and suggestions and, if necessary, made changes. After concurrence on numbers, rotation durations, and goals, we got approval from everyone. We were there. The only two things left to accomplish were to get the final two positions from surgery and hear the results of the committee.

The rumor mill was working and I heard that the committee had recommended a full department for us. Called in to see the dean, I was prepared. I knew we had won. I was not given a copy of the report. The dean told me that the chair of surgery had agreed to make us a section. Not a department. Since what I heard was only a rumor and the dean would not let me see the report, I felt I had no choice but to accept. It was one of my most serious mistakes, something I would regret for all time. But we had our residency, and on July 1, 1976, after much work by many people, our first two residents walked on the floor of the emergency department at DGH. The chief of surgery gave up the two positions; the program grew and exists today in a much expanded version.

Chapter XIX
Violence in the ED

As I said before, violence in the ED was not rare but not common. There were incidents involving patients, staff and visitors.

A patient drew a knife. The orderlies surrounded him, holding mattresses in front of their bodies so they wouldn't get hurt. One of the police officers assigned to us came into the room. In his mouth he had his pipe (yes, smoking was allowed!) and in his hand he had the biggest handgun I'd ever seen.

The officer casually pointed the gun at the patient and said, "I am counting to three. At that time, either you or the knife will be on the ground. I don't care which." The cop actually got to "two" before the knife clattered to the ground. The bad guy was arrested. He showed up the next night as a psych patient.

Crisis patient punched two visitors and one security guard in the face yesterday night report by ADO submitted.
Entry: 12/31/74
Floater: JMN
Violent psych patients were common.
Medical attendant JB bitten by patient last night.

Entry: 8/24/77
Floater: JMN
Pt. walked into triage area last P.M. with a rifle in a garbage brown bag. (No shooting)

Entry: 9/28/77
Floater: D.
Pt. with knife chasing another pt. Our security of no help. DPD called for help.

Entry: 10/03/77
Floater: JET
Attendant JK c/o bad human bite infection should be seen

Entry: 4/4/78
Floater: JNM
L.S. 8880642 –pt. is known manipulator who has been physically abusive—seen by psych last night and discharged—struck Dr. S. today and police have arrested him for A&B (Assault and Battery).

Entry: 11/27/78
Floater: BFB
On Friday, PF was hit by a big pt. Attendant sent home. Pt. was arrested by DPD for A & B.

Entry: 1/22/79
Floater: BFB

Most of the assailants weren't arrested. I wanted even the psych patients charged, but most of the time the police refused. I thought it was important to demonstrate that striking staff, docs or nurses, would not be tolerated. You shouldn't be crazy enough to hit your health care providers.

When I was a medical student rotating on psychiatry I had a black resident supervising me. He was the first, I believe resident in the University of Maryland history. We were called to the psych emergency room to see a patient. The patient was a paranoid schizophrenic. After a few minutes of conversation he hit the resident who immediately punched the patient out, putting him on the floor. "Don't ever get crazy enough to hit your doctor." I was impressed.

Chapter XX
Miscellaneous Incidents

There were incidents which occurred which were either not entries or just didn't fit together with others.

One night, during the winter holidays, I was pit boss. I had a black man as second in command. It was a cold blustery night, very typical for Detroit. The police had brought in a drunken police prisoner, white, with a scalp laceration, wearing only boxer shorts. The black resident went to sew him up. A few minutes later, he came to me. "Ron, can you sew this man up."

"What's the problem?"

"He doesn't want a black touching him."

"You know me better than that. I don't play that game."

"Ron, I am not making this drunk a civil rights issue. He is a drunken redneck and we have others to take care of."

So I went over, examined the cut and told him I would sew him up. He looked at me and said. "No kike is going to touch me. No kikes or niggers." I told him that's all we had, "kikes and niggers." I had him put out on the ambulance dock. I told the officer with him we were done with him. He was taken out on to the dock, in winter and snow coming down. The officer left him there for several hours; and brought him back. "He has something to say to you guys."

"I am really sorry. It won't happen again." We sewed him up.

One night, at DRH, I was called by a nurse because she couldn't insert a Foley catheter (a catheter inserted into the bladder for the purpose of draining urine) in a patient. When I went to the bedside I found an unconscious, elderly black woman, lying on the gurney with a gown on. The catheter tray was there all ready to be used. With the nurse's assistance, we spread her legs and I attempted to sterilize her vagina for the catheter insertion. When I started to wash her vagina she began moaning and moving her hips, as though she was having sexual intercourse. I stopped. All the nurse could say was, "Wow. It must have been a long time."

Once I was moonlighting at a small hospital. For me this involved covering the emergency room and the house. I was upstairs doing a work up, when a student nurse came to the nursing station. She had just removed a Foley catheter from a man who was now bleeding from his penis. The charge nurse told her to hold the penis very tight to see if compression would stop it. I went in after a few minutes to see how it was going. There stood the student holding this man's penis, when in a drunken stupor he said, "Not now honey, not now."

I was on duty one evening at DRH, shortly after we opened, when two EMT's came in with a big smile, and stopped right in front of me with a patient in a wheelchair. "What's going on, guys?"

"Guess where we picked this man up, sleeping it off. In a nice warm place."

"I'll bite, where?"

"Your old office at DGH. He was sleeping there. Security called. We thought we'd bring him here for continuity of care."

Rx (prescriptions) for Dilaudid is being forged using the names & narc #'s of Krome & K. These are definitely phonies as verified by Ralph—a rather amazing story—a phony drugstore called this AM to verify the narc #'s but no info given Police notified.
Entry: 1/8/75
Floater: JET

Forged prescriptions were not uncommon. At least in this case we were called. Eventually, two different prescription forms were developed; one for controlled substance; one, for non-controlled.

Commissioner R...Serious contamination in Burn Unit with 2 deaths and 1 septicemia. Temp. closed. He doesn't want to cut off ER for burns—so temporarily told ADO to clear all burn unit admissions with Dr. I. Burn Chief who plans now to switch burns to 2-2.
Entry: 1/27/75
Floater: JET

Contamination of any critical care unit was bad news. The origin could be from a staff member or a patient, and required movement of uncontaminated patients out and heavy duty washing and cleansing of the unit.

Brace yourself here comes a good one
Family of NG pt. #335018 came to ER to report that case of pt's lost or stolen partial plate has been solved—the searcher didn't do it after all. Seems as if the pt. swallowed her own partial plate into her hypo pharynx. Then reported same as missing or stolen. Then c/o sore throat –partial plate was found lodged in throat.
Entry: 8/24/75
Floater: JMN

Although our staff was frequently accused of stealing from patients—money, clothes—this was a first. And we didn't even do it!

Dr. A...from poison control called to say 12# of poorly cut PCP is on street of Detroit. Stuff is apparently heavy with cyanide.
2. Have talked to pharmacy for cyanide kits (amyl nitride) for standby use. 3. Talked to room 6 doc who subsequently informed staff.

Entry: 11/4/76
Floater: JNM

Drug abuse ran rampant in Detroit, as it did in a lot of other cities. We were lucky since we had good relations with the poison center and they shared information with us, frequently in advance of our actually seeing cases.

Took several veterans out to lunch today (Ron couldn't go—that's ok –he's always out to lunch)
Entry: 11/11/76
Floater: JET

In fact, it was not uncommon for all—or a group of us—to go out for lunch on Fridays. No one who was working the floor went, but anyone that wasn't was invited. We most often went to Hamtramck, the Polish section of Detroit. There was a bar there we frequented, with an upstairs balcony. One Friday we went, and one of the docs was to meet us there.

I was sitting on the balcony when this doc came in and told him to get a drink and come up. He leaned over the bar and asked for a screwdriver; I knew what was going to happen. The bartender handed him a screw driver (a tool). He returned it to the bartender and said he wanted a drink. It was filled. No one laughed, except me.

One evening in the fall, at DRH, an angry, really pissed off, drunk left the hospital, walked down the ambulance ramp to the street. He got in his car, gunned it up, and came charging up the ambulance ramp, until he got to the door, made a sharp right turn. He drove through the glass doors into the lobby. Anger management was not his strong suit.

12 burn patients from WCJ (Wayne County Jail) 9 prisoners –3 guards 2 prisoners with 2nd and 3rd degree burns admitted to burn unit 5 others held for smoke inhalation observation
Entry: 11/30/76
Floater: Krome

This was only a minor incident. We didn't even activate our disaster plan. But it certainly made for a stimulating day.

Mrs. H...was sad because we forgot her birthday on May 28. I told her we just took her out for her birthday. She said that was 1 year ago! (How come time goes by so fast even though I'm still so young?)
    Entry: 6/2/76
    Floater: JET

Not every thing in the ED was tragic and free of humor. Humor certainly made things easier. Patients could make us laugh; colleagues could make us laugh. In some, perhaps a lot, of incidents you had to see the humor or lose it. There was lots of crying and depression.

And occasionally there was forward movement, of one sort or another.

Many patients suffering from trauma are initially evaluated by E.Surg (Emergency Surgery—they handled all the trauma cases) team then often sent to multiple consultants for ultimate disposition. I feel that any pt. with) 1 consultations should be followed and discharged by E. Surg rather than left for the last consulting service.
    Entry: 6/13/76
    Floater: BFB

This was discussed with surgery and they made the appropriate changes in policy—a policy which still exists today.

Nursing home fire—1 pt. DOA 1 pt. 30% burns—initial report of many persons trapped, etc., Prompted us to clear Room 1 as temp. morgue—later situation facts did not support earlier fears.
    Entry: 2/25/77
    Floater: JNM

We had to rely on reports from the scene about the size of any disaster, or potential disaster. In those days, the call would go from the scene to fire dispatch, then to us. Dispatch wasn't always aware of what was going on at the scene.

Bizarre bizarre. Young white female council candidate picked up by Quinn floating naked on a raft in the Detroit River. Crisis center Dx no mental illness (just a showoff).
Entry 9/13/77
Floater: JET

Father Quinn was a unique man and priest. He was a fixture at DGH and in Greektown. I am not sure where his church was, but I do know that he was there when I started my internship. He was a recovering alcoholic and really took a lot of our drinking patients under his wing. He had a refurbished 1920s fire engine in beautiful shape and could be found patrolling the downtown streets of Detroit where he picked up down and out drunks. Often he would bring them to us. Equally he would take them to Sacred Heart Rehabilitation Center.

When it was slow on the streets, he would come and make rounds in the ED. He would go behind a curtain and see the patients we asked him to see. He could be heard chastising the patient, yelling and finally they would both come out and mount the fire engine, and go to Sacred Heart. He died years later.

Across the street from us, maybe a block away was a church. The priests would volunteer to help our patients in a variety of ways, or come over at the request of patients and their families. They often showed up to perform last rites; even when the patient was not Catholic. Once while I was operating on a patient who had sustained massive trauma, I looked up and saw one of the priests at the head of the operating table giving last rites. "Father, we might have a chance here. Gives us a break."

"It never hurts, son, to be prepared."

RN's on strike—ED RN's, however, are here! Sounds like a blow in favor of professionalism at last! Most appreciated.

Statement above short-lived. AM RN staff called in sick.
Closed hospital to all code 2 cases except Room 14 walk-ins.
Called EMS to this effect. Dr. Krome and Mr. H...notified.
RN staff redesigned for skeletal coverage.
Entry: 8/12/77
Floater: JMN

We lived in fear of strikes. RN's, LPN's medical attendants had unions and all of them could go out. Separately or together. Contracts were re-negotiated every three years. But who knew what would happen in the interim.

In the early days of our residency, we recruited hard for good people. We got candidates from all over the country. I often worried about the culture shock that would come to candidates from rural areas; those who never experienced urban living. I was more often wrong in my assumptions than right.

We had recruited and signed a nice, quiet young man from western Canada. He had never seen anything like Detroit, or DGH. He was working one night in our trauma room. I think it was even his first night. He was in the process of anesthetizing the patient's cut on his face. The patient hauled off and hit the resident in his face, cutting his nose. The resident required suturing. What an introduction to DGH.

H.S...937041 brought here by police as a psych, allegedly for campaigning for Mayor Young. Police wouldn't fill out papers. So nursing staff got suspicious—-it was all harassment.
Entry: 9/13/77
Floater: JET

This was recorded in the log. But I can't swear to the truth of it. Mr. Young wasn't popular with the police, among others, so they certainly could have done it.

We provided care to a number of politicians. For one mayor we were on-call if something happened at the city-county building. And we did respond. There was one councilman, well known for, among other things, his ability to consume alcohol. One night he was brought in injured, I am not sure from what. In the course of the work up a blood alcohol was obtained. A couple of days after he was treated, he called the hospital director complaining about his treatment, and threatened to go the press. I reviewed his chart, and informed the director that if he did, we would have to release his medical records in our own defense. This would include his blood alcohol level. The councilman backed off.

Coleman Young, long term mayor of Detroit, was a strong individual with great political strength. The press had a field day with him, but he did some good things for the city. He truly integrated the police and fire departments. Whereas, for generations promotion in the fire department was virtually entirely based on seniority, Mr. Young changed all this; and he imposed affirmative action in the police department. Both became more of a reflection of the population of Detroit.

On the other hand, most of his appointments were based on cronyism. And he had a unique way of antagonizing the white establishment, often, it appeared to me, in an attempt to improve the morale and self esteem of Detroit and its inhabitants. He decried any chance of regional government and mutual aid with the surrounding counties (largely white). Although Detroit had been polarized for decades, Mr. Young reinforced it. His antagonizing of the white establishment made him a hero to the blacks of Detroit.

This was, of course, unless it worked to the advantage of Detroit. I cannot embellish this more, since my memory lacks the knowledge of specific events.

He had his own doctor, a cousin, who was at Mr. Young's beck and call, and this relationship influenced later decisions relative to DRH/DGH. I remember one columnist who really took after him. In article published as we were negotiating closure and a new hospital, he had sarcastically, Mr. Young in our ER as the medics were bringing a patient in while they were doing CPR. "What's his problem?" Mr. Young asked. "Cardiac arrest." Pause, then Mr. Young said, "Don't forget to read him his rights."

In the late '60s, we instituted a renal transplant service. Getting donors, a problem now was even worse then. So the service used some cadaver kidneys, and a few donated by the victims of trauma. Whenever a kidney was harvested from a black person, and given to a black renal failure patient, it made the media and we were accused of using blacks for experiments. When the donor kidney was placed in a white patient, regardless of the kidney source, we were accused of treating whites preferentially. We couldn't win for losing.

Very busy morning—2 arrests in room 6.
Entry: 9/15/77
Floater: BFB
4 arrests room 6 yesterday 3 successful resuscitations
Entry: 9/16/77
Floater: JET

Sometimes we did things right. Or God stepped in to care for drunks and fools. You had to be one or the other.

DS woman, multiple lacerations, bruises, GSW (gun shot wounds). DOA, Brutal slaying
Entry: 8/16/77
Floater: JMN

Brutal slayings were not rare. Kids killing kids. Drive by shootings. One time EMS brought us the body of a patient who really belonged in the morgue. He had been cut in half. Horrible. When I was an intern, the police brought in a couple who were driving in a convertible small car. They had slid under a tractor trailer and been decapitated. Their heads were in the back seat.

Early Sat. A.M. a 38 y/o psych was transferred to DPI (Detroit Psychiatric Institute) & arrested upon arrival. Was brought back to DGH-DIE. In the process, all other psychs in van with pt. escaped.

Entry: 11/13/77
Floater: JET

They may have been crazy, but they weren't stupid!

Prisoner pt. signed out AMA. Had 38 caliber gun in bra.
Entry: 12/5/77
Floater: BCW

Rare, but I once found a snub nosed 38 caliber pistol in a woman's vagina.

2 yr. old 279 blood alcohol. Transferred to CHM.
Entry: 12/21/77
Floater: Krome

I can't believe what we do to our kids. This was an inadvertent ingestion of alcohol. There had to be some lying around. This kid was lucky.

W.C. set his stretcher on fire 5:15 A.M. in ED
Entry: 11/24/78
Floater: JET

It just seemed like we couldn't keep an eye on our patients all the time. This was support for restraints.

Sometimes well meaning medical students released the patient. Sometimes it was an attending physician. At times we would find a patient with his hands in the pocket of another patient.

I admit that physical restraints were not humane treatment. Insane patients had been released from their chains in Paris two hundred years ago. We still used them.

Busy AM DPO (Detroit Police Officer) GSW abd (abdomen)— chest 10AM to OR doing OK many cops many reporters crowd manageable

Entry: 11/27/80
Floater: JET

When we were at DGH, we got mostly the bad guys and another hospital got the cops. Here things were different; we got the cops and the bad guys. We had to keep them separate, of course. And one cop brought almost the entire force. Family was shuttled into a quiet room. Press and media were given information outside the Department. Sometimes the mayor came too. Often the Chief came. Not all mayors showed up. Anytime we could control the crowd it was a significant accomplishment.

10:30 PM noted several city and county prisoners were missing from their shackles. One city prisoner recovered; 2 others not found.
Entry: 8/22/74
Floater: SK

At DGH, prisoners were shackled to their gurneys and guards were to be in close proximity to watch them. Obviously, this didn't work in a consistent fashion.

Also 1 prisoner escaped from Screening on afternoons sev prisoner probs: #1 police do not stay with patients all the time; #2 they chain them up in a ridiculous manner to table leg—all they have to do is lift the table; #3 this prisoner got into an I&D set and stole a scalpel
Entry: 1/17/81
Floater: JET

What we wound up doing in Screening was put a place on the floor where the shackles could be fixed. But there was still, from time to time, a prisoner escape; not from Screening.

There were, however, occasional incidents that lent themselves to humor, involving an escaping psych patient or prisoner. One such incident occurred in the '80s. For about twenty years we provided the medical care at the Detroit Grand Prix, run on Belle Isle, before that in the streets of the city downtown. My wife was certified emergency nurse who volunteered to work the Grand Prix. She worked one of the first aid trailers at the race.

It was Sunday evening, and the event was over. I was in a trailer used for the medical center, and she in the first aid trailer. I got a radio call to come down to the first aid trailer and found my wife had fallen out of the trailer and hurt her ankles—both of them. She was taken to DRH and x-ray confirmed that she had broken them both. While she was waiting for an orthopedist, she and her two sisters who were at the race were placed in the suture room, at one end of a long hall. This was a room sometimes used for VIP'S. She was stoned on the pain medication and her sisters were standing next to her. The whole family had been raised in Ontario, in a small town. Coming to Detroit was a culture shock; coming to DRH was a bigger culture shock.

Down the hall came a running six-foot-plus naked black man, entirely naked, being chased by one of the police assigned to us. My sister-in-laws were terrorized and tried to hide in the cabinets in the room. Needless to say, they were much bigger than the cabinets. Luckily, the police officer managed to tackle him before he reached the room. Talk about culture shock!

"War Games" today set up for docs and resident staff
Entry 3/4/81
Floater: JET
"War Games" film to be shown today
Entry: 3/5/81
Floater: JMN

Showing this film, clearly anti-nuclear, turned out to be a real controversial event. I got calls and visits from a number of staff, who thought we would stimulate an anti nuclear movement from staff. I was unaware of any staff in favor of a nuclear war. Many of the comments originated from the radiation staff, who wanted equal time to present the other side of the story. We gave them the time, but they convinced no one that nuclear radiation was safe.

1 DIE(Died in Emergency) hanging from WCJ (Wayne County Jail)
Entry: 4/1/81
Floater: Krome

We knew this would hit the media. We had no information other than he arrived from jail and died in the ED. But we did notify administration. Actually, hanging or attempted hanging wasn't rare, especially in the county or city jails.

Stab of chest—hemothorax—admitted
5 codes 4 made it 1DIE 1 stab of the heart
Entry: 6/16/81
Floater: Krome

A good day. The critical patients made it. We had done good work. About a month later, another good day. Trauma victims who had been stabbed in the heart were not all that rare. I had repaired about twenty-six in my time; none had died.

Stabs of the heart did much better than gunshots of the heart. There was much controversy over time about opening the chest in the emergency department. In the early years there wasn't much choice since only emergency physicians were there when the patient needed them. Patients who were moribund and had sustained a chest injury close to or in the proximity of the heart were taken directly to the resuscitation room as a Trauma Code 1. One doctor at the head of the bed quickly intubated the patient. Another two placed large bore IV's and ran in fluid rapidly. Blood was drawn for transfusions. The chest was washed quickly with antiseptic solution. No other preparations were done, except a nasogastric tube and Foley catheter inserted. An incision was made and carried down into the chest cavity and the heart examined, the hole in the heart was repaired making sure that the coronary arteries were protected. The incision was usually accompanied by an outflow of large volumes of blood. The patient was taken to the OR, chest closed and chest tube place.

Our track record with patients who had sustained such an injury was remarkably good. Almost all made it. Once when I was a senior resident on surgery, a junior resident and I were making rounds in the recovery room. A patient who had his chest opened in the emergency room after he had been stabbed in the heart was still there. The junior resident had done the surgery. I introduced the patient to the doctor and told the patient that this was the doctor who saved his life. All the patient said was "cool." Nothing else. Our record was so good, that there repeaters, survivors of a stab who returned, later, with another one. It gave us good follow up.

Some staff wanted the chest opened in any moribund patient, even those who had no trauma. But this never got approved as a policy. There were patients who had their chests opened when they had sustained abdominal trauma and were moribund. In these cases, the aorta was clamped in an attempt to stop bleeding into the abdomen. Sometimes this worked.

One afternoon, when I wasn't even working the floor, EMS brought in a patient with a chest wound who was moribund. He was taken to the resuscitation room. I was fully dressed in civilian clothes when I went in and opened his chest. I had on a disposable gown, but the blood poured out and all over me. I was up to my elbows in his chest and his blood. When I heard the door open, I looked up. My senior son was brought over by SB to see his dad work. He never went in to medicine.

9 codes (7 saves)
Entry: 7/9/81
Floater: Krome

It was one of those days when we could hardly catch our breaths between codes.

Chapter XXI
Closure

In June 1980, Detroit General Hospital closed, marking the end of an era; no, the end of an epoch. When I started, I was told I'd be the first senior resident in the new hospital. It didn't happen! Detroit General was a significant financial drain for the city, never making money, or breaking even. Losing more every year. Detroit wanted out of the hospital business, at least the Mayor did.

There had been a long term commitment to move DGH to a new hospital at a new site, one closer to the other hospitals—Children's Hospital; Hutzel Hospital; Harper Hospital; Detroit Rehabilitation Institute— in the Medical Center. I don't know where or how the concept of a medical center originally started.

In 1976, things finally started to move. Planning began for the new hospital. Inpatient services requested the beds they wanted, in a best case scenario. The surgical services decided the number of operating rooms. Another group met to help plan the intensive care units. Each group met with consultants, who had the data to support decision making. In 1978, the mayor formed a new task force to start looking at shared services with the DMC.

A representative of the ED was on each planning group. In addition, we helped plan for the location of the operating rooms and intensive care units in the hospital. And, of course, we planned the ED.

The ED planning team consisted of residents, attendings, nursing staff, nursing supervisors, and administrative and clerical staff. Planning was a long, tedious process. There was the problem of patient privacy. The more open the ED, the more efficient and flexible its use. But the more open, the less privacy. We designed eight bed units (modules) with walls between the units so there was some semblance of privacy. We picked the location of radiology (with the radiologists); the laboratory (with their people); the pharmacy (with the pharmacists); the decontamination room (with the radiation people); and the resuscitation room. I wanted it up front, near the entrance. The surgery chief wanted it in the back so the codes would not be seen by people in the triage waiting area. There was much haggling, but the consultants openly told me, he had more power than I, and the resuscitation room was where he wanted it. Over the years it worked out alright. One thing I found most upsetting and frustrating was the layout of the ED. Certain units could not be where we wanted them because the architect said air shafts and the like had to be there. Here we were, not even a hole dug, and things had to be in a pre-determined location.

There was a pseudo-commitment for DRH to become the emergency unit for the entire medical center. The ARC (Ambulatory Reception Center) was to handle patients with relatively minor problems, and for private physicians to meet their patients. It consisted of multiple single rooms, with one outfitted as an eye room, and another for prisoner patients, and all with gynecology tables. We planned what went into the modules; the supply rooms; utility rooms, etc.

The design lasted twenty years before it was changed. Some things had to be fixed shortly after we moved. We didn't plan write up areas for the nursing staff in each module. When they were built, the doctors began using them, making for much crowding. The second error was our failure to put in enough sinks in the modules for staff to wash their hands; not corrected until the major reconstruction in 1980s. one would think that an adequate number of sinks would have been a critical part of the planning process.

An equipment list for the department was made after consulting with representatives of the chiefs of departments. Among the stuff ordered were portable defibrillator-monitors. We ordered sixteen, with the appropriate accessories; not cheap. No one questioned our order. Two years later when we moved into DRH, all the warranties had expired. We had to plead with the vendor to extend the warranty one year.

While all of this was going on, the politics were cooking. Laws had to change; agreements had to be made; complicated agreements involving many political and nonpolitical bodies and institutions. There were driving forces behind the changes and the vision of DRH becoming an integral part of the DMC. As I already implied, the dream had begun in the early '60's. I have avoided using real names; it is hard to even allude to history of this period without mentioning some key players.

Looming over all the dreams was the reality imposed by the economics of the late '70s, and the driving desire of Mayor Coleman Young to rid the city of the financial burden of the hospital. Mr. Young was a dominant political figure in Detroit. He almost always got what he wanted. And he wanted to rid Detroit of Receiving Hospital. Mr. Young had a background in labor unions and in the state legislature.

Another imposing, dominant figure in this change was Dr. Alexander Walt, Chairman of Surgery at Wayne State and chief of Surgery at the adult DMC hospitals. He was a man who walked the walk and talked the talk. He was the one who recruited me and was my chief for a number of years. Dr. Walt's vision was the complete integration of the DMC hospitals, with DRH being the principle, if not sole, emergency hospital. Dr. Walt's concept was that all emergencies for the DMC, except children, would enter DRH's Emergency Department and be admitted to other hospitals, based on the desires of the patient, the patient's doctor, and the availability of beds. The concept required that the patient be stable for transfer, and that all DMC's staff be admitted to practice at DRH. All children, younger than thirteen, would continue to go to CHM for emergencies and for admission. This had few supporters and lots of detractors. Some felt that DRH would preferentially admit patients to keep the beds occupied with insured patients, to the detriment of the other DMC hospitals. I am sure, whether it was said publicly or not, that the other hospital medical staffs didn't want their private patients to be in the bed next to druggies, alcoholics, or prisoners. Once they raised the concern that their patients would wait too long to be seen, even though we had data which showed that the wait at other DMC hospitals exceeded that at DRH.

Another key player was John Danielson, president of the DMC, who subsequently died, unrelated to his job. He was diligent, hard working, and a very pleasant man who had his eye on the vision of a united DMC. Mr. Danielson worked to establish the concept of a true DMC, working cooperatively together for the common good.

In 1981, Edward Thomas became the boss of DRH Hospital. This was after the move, but his work certainly did much to help unify the DMC, and drive DRH forward. He is a kind, gentle man who loves golf and poker. Mr. Thomas certainly strove to put DRH on sound financial footing. Some of what he did was successful; some wasn't. He made peace with the unions and we were free of union discord when we moved in, despite the fact that several had taken legal action to stop the closure.

In the background, through all of this was Les Bowman. He is a quiet unassuming man, who worked diligently for DRH. Although he had little to do with the physical move, he had much to do with the forward movement of DRH, and thus, DMC.

I am not sure why I include these people by name, and am sure I have left others out who contributed to these confused times. But it is hard to write about this very significant event, the transfer of ownership without including them.

The game plan went about like this. All current employees, all of them, received job offers to move to DRH, at their existing salaries, which were much higher than existing salaries in the DMC. Their salaries would be "red circled," frozen at that level until similar salaries came up to the "red circle" level. Health benefits and retirement benefits were lower, but each employee would keep their City retirement benefits. One could retire from DGH and DRH and have both. Of course, employees could refuse the job offer and stay with the City, but not necessarily in their current position. Those employees who went to DRH had a time limit when they could choose to return to the City; I don't remember how long. Many chose to go; many to stay. The transition of employees and the job offers were handled by the Personnel Officer, Pat Greaves, who I became close to over the years, both socially and otherwise. He would become vice-president of human resources at DRH. He was bright, articulate, and creative.

The plan was to close DGH and open DRH three to six weeks later under different ownership. This would allow for the ownership change to occur. It would also allow, although others will deny it, for a change in the unions. The time sequence and change in ownership meant the unions in existence at DGH would not be present at DRH until union elections, a very complex procedure, had occurred. However, the powers that be, recognizing that union disruption could be a bad thing, made a deal, which I am sure would be denied today, that the union would be recognized at DRH if they kept the peace. In addition, there would only be one union, with an increased membership. There was peace. I remain unsure of the legality of this procedure that by-passed both a NLRB vote and a union election ballot.

Mayor here for press conference
Entry: 2/8/80
Floater: BCW

The process had begun. The Mayor's press conference, held in a small auditorium at DGH, was to announce that the change was going to occur, and that the City was not abandoning the poor of Detroit. Later, when the city council passed the enabling legislation, that transferred hospital ownership, this was part of the transfer agreement, i.e., DRH would continue to see uninsured and underinsured patients.

Contingency planning for closing the hospital on April 15th. *Began today. Ron in meetings @ 8A, 11A, & 4P*
   Entry: 3/31/80
   Floater: BCW

The days were filled with meetings, and much of the subject material was repetitive and redundant. We weren't going to make an April deadline or even a May deadline. It was going to be June at the earliest.

We are in an advanced state of planning for closure in 12 days. Our patients are to be distributed to other DMC hospitals: Trauma to Harper; Med to Hutzel
   Entry: 4/3/80
   Floater: BCW

Things were not ready yet and the transfer of patients was not going to start yet. Morale was in the toilet. New equipment was impossible to get. Repairs took far more time than in the past. Absenteeism was starting to increase as employees burned their unused personal days and vacation time. Things were bad and getting worse.

The union filed an appeal.
   Entry; 4/15/80
   Floater: BCW

As predicted. It was denied. But it didn't add to morale.

P.... jailed in sit in last PM.
   Entry: 4/15/80
   Floater: BCW

Some staff honestly believed that a change in ownership was bad for the hospital, and bad for the city. The poor would suffer enormously from this change. The poor people's hospital was going to close! Some of our employees were so committed to preventing this change in ownership that they participated in sit-ins and other protests. Some were arrested and one was P...., who spent a night in jail for her beliefs.

There was a great deal of anxiety and apprehension among all employees and medical staff. Employees were concerned for their jobs and pay. Rallies in the evenings were held at a variety of churches and parks. Tempers were short and emotions ran high.

On April 16, 1980, the Detroit City Council approved the transfer, as a lease, to DMC. On May 21, 1980, specific plans were drawn up to phase out all wards. Inpatients were transferred to other DMC hospitals. Admissions were closed and only critical patients, who could not be transferred, were admitted.

The April deadline came and went. Admissions were curtailed. Morale continued an ever increasing downward spiral; broken equipment continued unrepaired. New equipment was only ordered if it was going into the new hospital. Existing equipment that could be used in the new hospital was marked to be moved, everyone praying for no more break downs.

In May, wards started to be phased out, patients to move to other hospitals identified. On June 9, the Department of Medicine stopped admitting patients. On June 11, CCU (Cardiac Care Unit) was closed. On the twelfth, SICU (Surgical Intensive Care Unit) was cut back to three beds. By the eighteenth, the ED was closed and the hospital empty. The plan was that the new hospital would open the next morning, for business. This didn't happen either. For about two to three weeks, the new hospital would remain closed. This produced lots of problems for a variety of people. First, we would have to have security through out the building. Secondly, since we were the primary response hospital for the Detroit paramedic units, we had to keep emergency physicians to answer the radios. No cafeteria open. Only security people. No televisions. Using gurneys as beds. Our emergency physicians stood ready at the radio. They were volunteers.

On June 18, the last patient left DRH and the hospital closed. Very emotional for us. The lighted sign outside the ED was taken down and given to me. I placed it and black and white pictures, showing scenes from the old hospital, on the walls in the new conference room.

The day we opened DRH there was a press release and TV showed up; so did a number of patients, who waited in line outside the ambulance doors, the entry to the new ED. I notified EMS dispatch that we were open for business. And at 12:30 p.m. we opened the ambulance doors. The first patient was a woman whose sole reason for coming was to be first; she was.

Chapter XXII
The Opening

The day we opened, there was a line up of patients waiting. Their first stop was the triage desk where they were met by the triage nurse, and assigned a treatment area. At registration they were entered into the computer. The chart was printed. Then things went downhill. We got off one chart, and then the computer failed. On the first day, I was scheduled on-call for trauma, but there was so much to do in the ED, I gave up the trauma call to a surgeon.

There were problems all over the place. Nothing we planned was working. The intercom system, wasn't working. We didn't have a list of stations. We weren't even sure how many had been installed. The HEAR radio which was needed to tie DRH to the state wide EMS system was still at DGH.

In OCU, the monitor wasn't hooked up at the nurse's station. There were no cubicle curtains there, or in various places in the Department. So much for privacy! We were supposed to have a ring down phone connecting us to the Detroit Renaissance Center, so security could alert us when they brought us a patient. And, of course, the ice machines in OCU and at the main nursing station weren't working. We had six crash carts; none of them stocked yet.

The phones in Screening didn't work right, they blinked but didn't ring.

There was a vacuum tube (pneumatic tube) system that connected the ED to the lab. It also connected to the clinics and other places. Lab requests and samples were placed in a plastic container, shaped like a rocket, and sent to the lab by entering the appropriate code. This system failed more often than it worked for the first several years. We had to hire couriers to take the lab specimens and bring back results. Using couriers was time consuming and expensive. Years after the move, the vacuum system was being blown out in an attempt to make it more reliable. Numerous samples which never got to their destination, some years old, were found.

By the time we moved in, many of the light bulbs were burned out. It took a long time to get replacements. The sprinkler system hung down from the ceiling so that a suicidal patient could use it to hang himself. They had to be fixed.

The satellite ED pharmacy was designed and built open—a clear violation of state law. It had to be built (rebuilt) enclosed, with walls and a locked door.

In Screening, in addition to the phone problem, lights were missing and there was no phone hook up for the EKG machines. There were no soap dispensers in Screening.

After a week, this is the summary of the problems:
– phones not ringing in Screening
– ice machines not working
– desk top copier not in
– EKG phone jacks in Screening
– prisoner holding sprinklers are not flush
– open pharmacy
– cubical curtains in OCU
– stapler and paper clips in Screening
– ashtrays in lobby
– ashtrays in psych
– ashtrays in x-ray
– 2 lights for laceration room
– 1 light for POD 1

– psych hamper bags for linen
– psych carpet needs to be removed
– psych rheostat for lights
– no staff are recording LMP (last menstrual period) and allergies
– eye box not complete
– crash carts need to be equipped and supplied

Quite an impressive list and that doesn't include the policies which needed rewriting, or the new ones that needed writing. Oh, and, of course, of the two x-ray rooms, we were lucky to have one working.

Pneumatic tubes down all weekend lab running 3-4 hrs. behind
   Entry: 7/14/80
   Floater: JMN

Perhaps the most complicated problem to work with was the pneumatic tubes which often went down and required couriers. And on weekends there was no one available to repair it anyhow. Years later, when the tubes were being blown out, a lot of material was found in the clinic. So much for high tech.

And when the computer went down, the registration personnel had to do charts by hand. Then later, when the computer came up, all the data had to be entered.

Slowly, over time DRH opened more and more beds. The ED census began to increase.

Chapter XXIII
Cold Exposure

Cold exposure DIE in Room 4
Entry: 01/09/77
Floater: JET

As temperatures fell, the number of people with cold exposure increased, as the number of homeless increased. Frostbites were common and deaths, not unusual. The homeless slept on the streets in their cardboard houses, sometimes on hot air vents; sometimes with newspapers as blankets; sometimes under bridges. Many did not have gloves or even shoes, allowing frostbite to occur. Alcohol ingestion may have made the homeless feel better, but did not protect from exposure.

Almost every morning, early, or late at night, EMS would roll in with someone who had prolonged cold exposure. Patients with frostbite would wander in during the day, not detecting the frostbite until they had pain, or noticed the skin changes when they went to the shelter in the evening, and got undressed. There were, and are, lots of shelters open in Detroit for the homeless, regardless of age. But they had to be there by early evening and leave by early morning. Some provided meals.

Cardiac arrest in a hypothermic patient required prolonged

resuscitation; they had to be warmed until they reached a core body temperature level sufficient to sustain cardiac activity.

When an exposed patient came in, a heating blanket was placed on the gurney, under the patient. A warm blanket covered him, and IV's with heated fluids was given rapidly. The fluids were kept in a warmer until used. If the patient's response was sluggish, or non-existent, a nasogastric tube was placed and warm or hot saline run into his stomach and sucked out. Heated, humidified oxygen was administered.

Different methods for heating the patient were developed and tried. Sometimes the left chest was opened and warmed saline washed right over the heart and major vessels. We even tried cardiac by-pass and running in heated blood. If there was no heart beat, a thumper, an external device used to provide continuous external massage, was used. This process could go on for hours, tying up staff and the room.

Wm. A. SICU (Surgical Intensive Care Unit) admitted hypothermia & frostbite
Entry: 1/12/82
Floater: JET

Double header. Cold exposure squared; but he made it,

Wm. David #26378 was discharged at 7AM today and ran out of the hospital with only a gown on and then jumped thru window of medical records-back in restraints—-evaluation continues.
Entry: 1/26/77
Floater: JNM

A rare, but not uncommon, event. Once, during the Detroit riots, the Army was assembling in the street right in front of the hospital, when an ED patient jumped out of the window. He only had a gown on, no shoes or slippers. An IV line was dangling from his arm. He was in DT's. The Army guys surrounded him, pointing their M-16's at him. All of us yelled at the Army. The patient sobered up very quickly. He returned to the ED.

Once, a psych patient escaped and ran up the stairs. He jumped from a fourth floor window and had to be resuscitated on the street.

There seems to be a constant heating/cooling imbalance in the ED. Is this an insurmountable engineering problem?
Entry: 2/1/77
Floater: JNM
So hot in 6/7/8 and so much decrease in water, patients are getting dehydrated
Entry: 5/30/78
Floater: Krome

The problem with the heat and cooling was a prolonged one. We found out later that the wiring was backwards! So in the summer we got heat; in the winter, cold. Typical city operation.

Tanker explosion—auto accident on freeway. Pt. brought in with 3rd degree burns face and hands. Scalped.
Entry: 2/7/77
Floater: BFB

It was a mess. Chaos, controlled chaos, ruled. IV's were started. The scalp tacked back on. Antibiotics started. And tetanus toxoid given. Pain medication was given.

There was a witnessed arrest in OCU early this AM.— Advanced Life Support went well—complexes returned stat but pt. is comatose. In addition, RN staff reported that Mrs. P...(RN) O.C.U. may not have functioned up to standards during the initial phases of the resuscitative effort—RN staff to look into the matter and report subsequently.
Entry: 2/23/77
Floater: JMN

The nurse was reprimanded and went back to an ACLS course. But the patient made it and that's all that counts.

Chapter XXIV
Our Bad

It is always tough to write, or even admit there were mistakes, system errors or people errors. And the patient paid; either by getting sicker, or dying, or having a non-lethal complication. Overall, ninety-five percent of patients who arrived alive left alive.

Pt. IT seen here 12/14/74 for chest pain and D/C ed by med res. Returned in C-arrest 12/16/74 & expired. Case already discussed with med res
   Entry: 12/16/74
   Floater: JET

The diagnosis of myocardial infarction was difficult in those days; even now it is not always easy. The use of cardiac markers was limited. The most reliable indicators were the changing EKG and a suspicious mind. No doubt it would have been better to keep this patient for a prolonged period.

Pt. LR. 92847 referred to medicine—found by nursing staff this A M to have an oral endotracheal tube in place with a cuff deflated, emesis in trachea and no humidification on tube. Cuff

inflated humidification on tube. Cuff inflated, humidification applied, trachea suctioned and medical resident informed.
  Entry: 6/18/76
  Floater: BFB

In this case, whoever intubated the patient wasn't keeping an eye on him or notifying the nursing staff. The patient, and we, were lucky.

CN blunt trauma to abd—acute abd missed. Pt. sat about 12 hours without IV, NG (nasogastric tube), and without bloods being drawn. Triaged to Room 6 by triage nurse per DPD run slip.
  LA 902353 initial Dx DT's –obvious lt. hemiparesis missed Pt. here about 16 hours went to angio 6/20 AM. Had no NG tube in.
  EG—subdural hematomas—was not stabilized properly. Was comatose and decerebrating. No NG tube, no airway. Had respiratory arrest in main x-ray and aspirated all over the place.
  Entry: 6/20/76
  Float: JET

Each of these cases demonstrated a careless approach by a moonlighter, someone who didn't know what he should have known.

Iatrogenic pneumothorax pt. DH
  Entry: 6/1/77
  Floater: BFB

Over time, medicine, emergency medicine, changed. Central venous lines were an important method of giving IV fluids, or monitoring their volumes. We had long IV catheters which could be inserted peripherally and threaded into the superior vena cava. But it was difficult to give large volumes rapidly. Venous cut downs were used to insert large bore catheters and thread them up. These took time to do and insert. Then came other forms of insertion of large catheters. Prime among these were the subclavian lines, to run a catheter directly into the subclavian vein and into the superior vena cava. But it was, and is, not free of complications, usually a pneumothorax (air in the chest). Consequently, a chest x-ray after insertion was necessary. Then chest tube insertion and admission. Regretfully, in our hands it wasn't uncommon to have a complication. At least once, I had to meet with the chief of medicine, since medicine had most of the admissions.

Pneumo secondary to subclavian in room 4 last nite
Room doc did not make rounds this AM- and about 12:30 PM a young lady was found in CP arrest (Cardio-pulmonary arrest). She subsequently died, after getting bilateral pneumo from subclavians.
Entry: 8/24/76
Floater: JET

I had sent out numerous memos about the necessity of making rounds with their relief, patient by patient. It was obvious that not everyone did it. In this case the patient paid for our double error—with her life.

Not all bads were without humor.

"Disaster" on Saturday about 5 PM Phase III. Nobody called or paged me. Reason—only your name is on disaster list. Added Assoc Dir name and #. Also nursing station should have our home phones. Disaster was a phony—was sent from Cleveland- wrong radio frequency used.
Entry: 8/23/76
Floater: JET

I don't know what was going on in Cleveland, but I sure hope they got the message. I know we improved our disaster phone listing because of them. I didn't even know the radio would work that far!

H.M. had chest tube inserted in abdomen—is scheduled for OR.

Entry: 11/25/77
Floater: BFB

If the appropriate procedures were followed, this shouldn't have happened. Chest tubes belong in the chest, not the abdomen.

LW intubated with stomach full of activated charcoal—vomited—admitted with possible aspiration pneumonia.
Entry: 10/16/78
Floater: BFB

I am sure she aspirated. This was a clear no-no in treatment. The doc should have known better.

Incident reports—AC 407453 wrong blood hung up
Entry: 8/18/80
Floater: JMN

This patient had been admitted to the ED as an UGI (Upper Gastrointestinal) bleeder. Although she required blood transfusions, she didn't require the wrong blood. Usually each unit of blood was triple checked before being given to a patient. Obviously, this wasn't done here.

Chapter XXV
Rape

Rape counselor reports that pt. PM 925768 case should be reviewed to see if Rx procedure employed was justified.
Entry: 2/24/77
Floater: JMN

I am not sure when the rape counseling service started. They came from the DPD. In the beginning they were volunteers; then, full time employees. This was a needed service for us and for our patients

We saw lots of rape victims. One year we saw over 1500 rape victims. In the beginning, the police wanted the patients seen by the gynecology resident on duty. But we came to an agreement that emergency physicians would see the patients first and only refer them to gynecology if there was a problem. Treatment guidelines were worked out.

Not all victims were accompanied by a police officer; many came with family or by themselves. They were seen by an emergency physician, examined, had specimens and blood taken. Then, they saw the rape counselor. If a police report was not made, the rape counselor arranged it.

Every rape victim was given venereal disease prophylaxis using the most current Center for Disease Control guidelines. There was no treatment for herpes or AIDS. In addition, each patient, unless already pregnant, was offered an oral contraceptive. Of course, a positive test meant they were currently pregnant, and were not even offered oral contraceptive. All medications were discussed with the patient. The patients had the right to refuse all and any medication. The oral contraceptive was diethylstilbestrol. It had been used in pregnant women in the past and was associated with cancer of the cervix in female offspring of women who took it. The rape counselors were really pissed at our use of this drug. In their opinion, even the remote possibility of cancer out weighed its use.

Every precaution was taken to insure that the patient was not pregnant; it did have a one time use and not continual use. Finally pregnancy was rare as a result of rape; it happened, but was rare. In 1978, one of these rare events happened.

Pt. S.J. 947310 seen here 3-21-78 given DES prescription— had no money to get Rx filled—got pregnant. Had Ab (abortion) @ DGH 5-22-78. Plan: give out pre-packaged samples.
Entry: 7/27/78
Floater: JET

It happened but it was rare. We began dispensing it right in the emergency department.

The rape counselors weren't only pissed but wanted all use stopped. There were times, I admit, that a pregnancy test was missed, or a patient given the medication before the test came back. Physicians who allowed this to happen were disciplined. In addition, sometimes the rape victims waited an unconscionable period of time before coming in and reporting the rape. Few doctors liked doing these examinations; they all had to be reviewed and were followed sometime later with a court appearance. An event no one wanted.

The use of this medication provoked the case review. In fact, everything we did was by protocol. I am not sure why they were so against the use of diethylstilbestrol in these circumstances, but it was a sore spot between us. A problem that was constantly resurrected.

To make sure we had a good working relationship with the rape counselors, I in a sudden epiphany, appointed a woman doctor as liaison. It didn't work. The protocols developed and implemented were ok; but the use of diethylstilbestrol continued as a sticking point. Our differences only got worse. A member of Detroit City Council had taken the RCC under her wing. When things between us heated up, we got a request to appear before City Council; not really a request as much as a command. So three of us from DGH went; me; the lady who was liaison with RCC, and the hospital director.

At the meeting, a number of questions came up regarding how we handled rape victims. They asked for a lot of data, most of which we didn't have with us. She did. She had obviously been feed a lot of material by the RCC. But we went back, collected the data we thought we needed and returned about a week later to the Council meeting. We were, once again, subjected to a battery of questions. Included in this mess was the accusation that we were using an experimental drug (DES) to experiment on the patients; the victims of rape. While I took great umbrage at this, the hospital director sat there and never made a comment. He and I discussed his lack of action, but I don't really think he ever heard me. We continued doing what was right and nothing of any significance changed.

RCC problems: (a) pt. allegedly given DES although had no penetration—review of chart showed possible penetration—no change in therapy. (b) pt. allegedly had anal intercourse without proper rectal exam—review of chart shows both vaginal and anal intercourse with proper P.E.
Entry: 6/1/77
Floater: BFB

The disagreements between us and RCC were continuing and even escalating. The counselors were reading our charts, as they should. Instead of asking for clarification they raised flags at morning report. It was at the point that every error, or pseudo- error, we made was a major cause celebre.

Rape victims were not a rare occurrence in our Department.

There were weekends when we saw a couple dozen victims. Children victims of rape were seen at CHM. Data from the rape counseling center in 1977 showed we were seeing an average of thirty-five patients per week, and fourteen per weekend. Some of the rape victims were pathetic and suffered greatly at the hands of the assailant. Some were pregnant, far along; some were aged and were beaten before or after the rape incident. Some, however, were treated with courtesy, if being raped can be classified as a courteous incident; the assailant even wearing a condom.

Sgt. M...Sex crimes Division wants cop present during P.E...I spoke to Mr. H....we agreed that cop could talk to MD after PE complete.
Entry: 3/31/77
Floater: Krome
DES sheets have been re-stenciled 5000 in stock
Entry: 4/1/77
Floater: JET

DES information sheets were distributed to rape victims. This was followed by the development of a DES permit sheet, for patients to sign. More and more paper work.

There was no office space for the counselors in the ED at DGH. They did get some space on the eighth floor, but it really was not in a convenient location. So we arranged for them to use the back of Screening, an area which was used as a conference room. Consequently, privacy which they sought was not always found! And they frequently got bumped.

Rape in clinic pt. Tuesday 3 P.M.
Entry: 10/30/80
Floater: JMN

Even within the clinic during broad daylight, as busy as it was, the assailant managed to drag this woman into the restroom and rape her.

84 y/o woman rape victim
Entry: 11/19/81
Floater: Krome
19 rapes this weekend
Entry: 4/26/82
Floater: JET

I am not sure this was a record, but if it wasn't, it was very close. Rapes went up as the weather got warmer, and were more common on weekends than during the week. They were higher during holidays. In 1979, over the Christmas holidays we saw thirty-five victims; over New Years, twenty-two.

Many times mothers brought in their daughters, teenagers, for pelvic examinations, because they were concerned about possible sexual activity. There were times when they suspected rape had occurred. When they mentioned possible rape, we would get the counselor involved. In general we didn't do pelvic examinations without a clear indication, especially without the teenager's consent. This, on occasion produced a not so friendly confrontation. It was hard to convince mothers that his was not the best way to assess their daughter's sexual activity.

Nursing home and boarding home residents were also a peculiar problem. Frequently brought in by caregivers, often confused and/or disoriented, days or weeks after an alleged attempted rape, a clear history was almost impossible to gain. So we treated with STD prophylaxis, got a pregnancy test; never offered oral contraception. If they accused a staff member the case was turned over to social services.

Chapter XXVI
Equipment and Supplies

Broken equipment and missing supplies, or equipment, was not unusual. I can't begin to make a list because there wouldn't be room for anything else.

Mr. J. called 3 x's over 3 days to fix back doors—nobody has come
   Entry: 1/12/77
   Floater: JET

At DGH there was a set of swinging back doors that led to the ambulance entry. They were broken more often than not. We had to go to the level of the hospital director before we got them working. In the winter the wind, and sometimes snow, came whipping in to the ER.

There is an aside I must tell related to the doors. Prior to the Riot, when police didn't treat blacks well, they would put the prisoner on the gurney with his head extending over the edge, and use his head as a battering ram to open the doors. Gee, I wonder why the riots happened.

All bed pan steamer sterilizing devices are not operating—nothing in the department works

Entry: 5/23/78
Floater: JMN

Since we didn't use disposable bed pans, believe it or not, all bed pans were supposed to be sterilized and reused. When the sterilizers went down, a not unusual occurrence, they were hand washed and a sterilizing solution used. Another chore about which the nursing staff weren't happy. And it wasn't rare. Sometimes it was the bed pan washer.

Bed pain washer in OCU—will take 1 week to get parts.
Entry: 1/30/80
Floater: BFB
Sinks in room #4 plugged. Maintenance no response
Entry: 6/9/78
Floater: Krome

If it wasn't one thing, it was another.

No suction equipment has been checked—bottom line—25 units in department 12 work
Entry: 7/11/78
Floater: BCW

Suction units had an important use, but they had to work. They were never checked. We wound up ordering nineteen new units.

Laryngoscope missing from 7
Entry: 8/31/78
Floater: BCW

Pieces of equipment which could be sold on the gray market, or used by residents, nurse, or attendants would periodically turn up missing. Perhaps the most common were the suture sets; then laryngoscopes, and even Ambu bags. Medical students took suture kits so they could go home and practice.

Blood gas machines both busted in ER lab. Gases being done @ Memorial.
Entry: 9/15/78
Floater: BCW

This was a machine that had real meaning in taking care of patients. To have to go across the street to gain access was not only bad care, but also embarrassing.

Incubator in Room 8 not working—down for repair.
Entry: 1/3/79
Floater: BCW
Incubator broken—in maintenance
Entry: 1/31/80
Floater: BCW

No incubator. We could only pray for no births until it was repaired. You can see this wasn't that uncommon.

EKG machines still out.
Entry: 1/9/880
Floater: Krome

Even EKG machines were not immune from breakage. There were always prolonged periods before they would be back up. Sometimes it was just an electrode missing. Sometimes it was a major problem. It didn't matter; we didn't have back up supplies.

Our lamp order was overlooked by vendor—his price has gone up—we're using City Hall pressure to get them.
Entry: 1/16/80
Floater: JET

If we didn't screw things up, we could always depend on our purchasing department or the vendors themselves to help out.

Cox fracture last night had to get tongs from M. Carmel
We didn't have any
Harper couldn't lend us any
Entry: 3/13/80
Floater: BCW
There are about 5 sets in OR
Entry 3/14/80
Floater: JET

Sometimes we were our own worst enemies.

Missing electric blanket
Entry: 2/5/81
Floater: Krome

This wasn't the first time we lost an electric blanket during the season. Once before, housekeeping threw one out by mistake. Sometimes they were left on the gurney with the patient and wound up on the floor.

Out of urinals/bedpans
Entry: 2/29/81
Floater: Krome

Can you believe it? We were using metal bedpans and urinals, sterilized. How could we run out of them?

Elevators were broken on the weekend for about 4 hours. Pt from Harper was carried up 1 flight of stairs.
Entry: 3/24/80
Floater: JET

A brand new hospital and already the elevators were broken.

Chapter XXVII
Bump in the Night

During my internship, DGH provided at least the interns, room and laundry. We had to pay for our food. The laundry was done by prisoners in the Detroit House of Corrections. There was even money bet that you would get your own laundry back. The laundry markers were metal tags. You had to be very careful when you put on your underwear or socks.

The rooms given to interns were two-man rooms (there were no women in our internship class). But the powers were clever about it. Each room was assigned one single and one married intern. The concept being that the married intern would go home on his nights off, leaving the single intern with a room alone, at least thee out of four days.

We were housed on the eighth floor of a newer building. Nothing else was on the same floor. There was a common bathroom and a common shower with three shower stalls. And you had to go down the hall to use either. In the morning or in the evening there was a line up for the showers. One evening a colleague came into my room where several of us were bullshitting.

I remember him and the incident very well. He was wearing a big smile as he looked right at me and said, "Go shower." "Why?"

"Go see." So I went in to the shower room, where one stall was being used. "You going to be long, buddy?" A very feminine voice replied, "Not much longer." I went back to my room. "There is a woman in there!"

They all started laughing. Finally, the story came out. Some of it I know is factual; some I am not sure about. It seems as though, one of our interns was living in his room with a belly dancer from Greektown. His married roommate was an unwilling voyeur of this relationship. But no one said anything to the administration.

The story goes, and I won't mention his name because he is still around Detroit, that he had inherited this lady from a surgical resident. I don't think he inherited her as much as he was introduced to her. Once I saw him at the eighth floor elevator, dressed to the nines, waiting for an elevator so they could go out. This lasted almost the whole internship year. I asked him, once, what he said going to do when the year was gone. He had bought her a one way ticket to Chicago on a Grayhound bus. He went to Vietnam.

Although I haven't recounted them, there were a fair number of sexual trysts. Midnight rendezvous using linen closets were not uncommon, according to the scuttle butt. This has become an urban legend. But the nurses and other single women at the hospital had their standards. During my internship year, single lab and x-ray techs had a party every Friday night; you had to be single to attend. There was one nurse anesthetist who refused to sleep with any house officer, married or single. She would only go to bed with attending physicians; married or single.

I went to some and at one I got good and drunk. The party was on the east side of Detroit. By this time I had a room in a house on the west side. I had bought a brand new Triumph, TR3; the first car I had ever bought. Living in this home was a unique experience for me anyway. The house was owned by an elderly couple, who's daughter had just gone a way to college, and they rented me her room, which was actually the top floor of the house. No kitchen but otherwise it was like an efficiency apartment. The husband and wife hovered over me, frequently asking me if I had called my mother. The man used to tell me I could bring a woman home if I wanted; not something I even considered.

In any case on this night when I got so drunk, I drove home in my brand new car, across town, using the freeway system and moving at a good speed. I pulled into the driveway and went in and upstairs. I was washing up in the bathroom when I heard through the open window the unmistakable sounds of a car rolling. I knew. I ran downstairs and outside in my underwear and stood watching my car rolling out of one driveway into another. I stood watching until it stopped in the middle of the street. I got in and pulled it into my driveway, and pulled the brake and put it into gear. How it missed hitting everything was and is beyond me. Except, God takes care of fools and drunks.

At DGH, one evening the police brought in some men of Armenian extraction, who had gotten in to an altercation at the Dodge Main plant. It seems as though a man had hit on one of the Armenian women, and the rest of the clan had taken exception and an altercation had resulted.

The police brought in eight to ten of the warriors at the same time. They were all put in Room 4, the trauma room; there was only one who had been shot. He, who was shot, had only a grazing wound from a .22. The remainder had cuts and bruises. Nothing significant. Nobody spoke English, but they all managed to call each other the same thing, "mother fucker." It was the only thing that came out clearly.

"Mother fucker" was a very common expletive in the emergency department. I remember a student telling me he had asked a patient to call him, "Dr. Mother fucker" out of respect. One time I overheard one prisoner calling another mother fucker. The second replied that if he would keep his mother off the street, he wouldn't fuck her. Nice fight broke out.

One night the police had broken up a fight between two motorcycle gangs. There were a lot of chains, poles, and knifes. About ten to twelve total were involved in the two gangs. The police, of course, brought them all to DGH, where they met in the lobby, and immediately continued the fight. Chairs all over the place; yelling and swearing; pushing visitors. Staff stayed out of it, although some were tempted,

I'm sure. Eventually the cops cooled it down, and we proceeded to treat the injured. Another night in the city.

Once, a surgery resident and I were sitting at the write-up desk watching the action in Module 1 (the trauma module). It wasn't especially busy. He and I were discussing a case he was seeing. We decided we needed to create an "asshole scale" to categorize the various and sundry patients and drunks seen. Of course, it was based on signs of being obnoxious. We looked up and saw a prisoner patient talking to his mother. Suddenly the patient lashed out and hit his mother in the face. This was a ten. There could be none higher.

On June 11, 1982, Detroit had one of its biggest manmade disasters in many years. A lone gunman equipped with a shotgun and a firebomb went in to the Buhl Building up to the eighth floor, where he shot and killed a young receptionist, and wrecked havoc throughout the offices. An apparent paranoid schizophrenic, he apparently came to collect a debt from the lawyers housed there. Thirty-eight victims later, he was arrested. Two victims had jumped. The helicopter service was not functioning. I had radio communications with the scene, and managed to confuse things for the paramedics and dispatch. Five victims were taken to another downtown hospital. It was the only time a disaster had managed to overwhelm our resources.

In the early days of heart valve replacements, there was a peculiar valve used for aortic valve replacement. It was a ball valve; with a Teflon covered ball held in a cage made of three prongs of metal (I don't know what kind.). All the surfaces were covered with Teflon. When the heart contracted, the ball was pushed into the cage to the top. When the heart relaxed, the ball fell back to the base. There were plenty of complications. But the truly bizarre thing was when the ball went up to the top of cage it made a clicking noise, which the patient could hear as could those around him. Can you imagine lying in bed in the quiet of night listening to the constant clicking sound, know when it stopped, so did your heart! When these patients sustained a cardiac arrest, the first thing that had to be done was the chest had to be pounded to loosen the ball. I never saw any of these patients successfully resuscitated.

Chapter XXVIII
Time to Go

It was time to leave. I had to get out. I didn't want to die there and the happiness and joy were gone. When I started I was excited about going to work. I came in early and worked late. Each day brought new challenges. Now I was beginning to hate it, dreading every day. I had cried wolf so often, no one listened to me; no one even heard me. There were already rumors that I was going to leave.

I gave ninety days notice. When I did, a columnist heard about it and came to do an interview. Very flattering. In fact, we had contact when I was a resident. He had cut his finger tip off. A medical student threw the tip into the trash. I retrieved it, and sewed it back in place. It took. He never forgot it.

The interview took place in my office at DRH. Scattered around were boxes I hadn't even opened or bothered to empty. The bookcases had books on them and some plaques were up. But, in general, it looked exactly as it had when I came. It was as though I never took possession. He noticed and commented on it in his article. It was as though, he said, I looked at this move as a temporary thing; like I only paused at DRH, but was going to move one. I was there about four years before I left.

Moving from DGH to DRH brought a change in the environment,

not only in physical but also in attitudes. The comfortable feelings of DGH were gone. We went from being an urban, city-county hospital to a privately owned hospital. We had been king of the hill. Now we were second class citizens. The panacea that we all thought would occur when we moved to DRH never materialized. We were owned by the other DMC hospital, actually the DMC Corporation, leased from Detroit. The money given to start up was quickly burned to support some of the other hospitals. We quickly became a poor hospital. Although the cumbersome bureaucracy of the City was gone, it was replaced. Others controlled our destiny.

The concept of DRH being the main ED for the Center never came to fruition. Oh, there were meetings to discuss it, with junior administrators of the other adult hospitals. CHM was never considered. Hutzel, formerly Women's Hospital, was about two miles from us. So they used the argument of geography. Harper was about one mile away. There was a tunnel that connected DRH, Harper, and CHM, and patients could and did go back and forth. Whereas Hutzel had a geographical consideration, Harper didn't.

At the meetings the administrators forgot we hade the contract to provide emergency care at both, and at Grace-Sinai. So we had all the hard data. Claims that we were slower in providing care at Harper were not true; but the junior administrator lied and said DRH was twice as slow as Harper. And I confronted her outside the meeting. She immediately went to the administrator from DRH and complained. I never told him that I was so angry at her because she blatantly lied to him.

At Hutzel, we distributed a form to members of the medical staff asking how they wanted us to handle their patients. Six months later we did it again. We found more confidence in our emergency staff. When we moved into DRH, we did the same thing. But the entire Harper medical staff was not on the staff of DRH; so they never got the form. But it wouldn't have made any difference. Most didn't want their private patients seen there anyhow. Oh, they raised a variety of objections; crowding; prisoners; waits; etc.

And it worked. Some of the problems were generated by us. Over time we didn't call the patients' private doctor reliably. In time, Harper put money into their "urgent care center," as their emergency department was called. Hutzel closed and moved into Harper. Their emergency patients were seen in the urgent care center.

So went a vision some had since the 1960s. So went my vision.

Not only was I lied to by the junior administrators of Harper, but even at DRH there were some who lied too. Just out and out lied. One was a junior administrator in the finance department who I frequently dealt with regarding the ED finances. I won't mention his name here, and I am not sure he knows that I know. But it was disheartening; to say the least, that people who I had to rely on would so openly lied. I guess I was just too trusting.

Many employees went back to the city. They didn't like the freeze on their salaries. They didn't like the retirement plan. They didn't like the fact that a number of new staff came in over them. They didn't like the apparent veto power of Harper. Things were just not as comfortable at DRH.

There were other depressing things. Money was tight, and a contract was negotiated with the county for the treatment of uninsured and underinsured patients. Under this plan, patients covered by the county would be transferred to the county hospital. We had to call on each transfer, and the receiving hospital had the right to refuse. So what in fact happened was drug addicts, alcohols, and others with the complications, were refused, and "nice" patients, with socially acceptable diseases, were transferred. We became, in essence, a hospital for drug addicts and alcoholics and trauma victims! It was demoralizing and depressing.

I had an offer from a suburban, privately owned hospital. I had mixed feelings about leaving. I had grown up both professionally and personally at DGH and DRH. When I came there in 1961, I was fresh out of medical school. I married while I was there; I had three kids while there. I did my residency there. I rose in the academic arena while there. I had attained national recognition in emergency medicine while there. Everything I had done, I had done there. I owed big time dues to my colleagues there, and to the nursing staff and the other staff there. I knew virtually everybody there. The hospital spun around the ED. We had significant power in the system. We had lots of media coverage; some good, some bad. When Detroit was known as "Murder City," we even made national television. I did a news column on substance abuse. But things had changed.

I could not get the changes I felt we still needed. I had cried wolf so often no one was paying attention; no one was listening. My health was going into the toilet. I developed hypertension there, and psoriasis. I had gained weight and I smoked. I knew I had to leave.

On the other hand, the offer was good. It offered new challenges. The money was good and I could, again, do what I wanted. I was getting pressure to decide. I would get good money and have less stress and meet new challenges. I was dead at DRH. So I left. I was very depressed that I had to go.

I had to give three months' notice. During this time I made rounds and said goodbye to my friends, some of them of thirty years' duration. I cried and they cried. There were those who accused me of leaving because I didn't like blacks, alcoholics or druggies. There were those who thought I went just for the money. But there were also those who came to me and told me they understood and wished me well. I knew deep down that my successor would succeed where I didn't; he did.

I have no regrets. I fulfilled the objectives set out for me, by me, when I started, and then some. I was ready to move on. But what was most important, I did it my way, with little or no compromise with my ethics or ideals.

I believe that every teacher is best judged by the accomplishments of his students. Then on this basis, on the basis of my students, judge me. The four who were the core of Receiving during this golden age, and were, to some extent mentored by me, were (in alphabetical order):

Brooks F. Bock, MD, FACEP, currently president of Harper University Hospital, formerly president of both American College of Emergency Physicians and American Board of Emergency Medicine (separately); first residency director of emergency medicine residency Wayne State University School of Medicine and DRH; first chairman of the Department of Emergency Medicine, Wayne State University School of Medicine; physician in chief, emergency medicine, Detroit Medical Center, and floater, emergency medicine, DRH. **floater**

John N. Mehelas, MD, founder of the first EMT training course at DRH and Wayne County Community College. **floater**

Judith E. Tintinalli, MD, FACEP, former President of the American Board of Emergency Medicine (first woman president); former residency program director, Wayne State University School of Medicine; currently professor and chairperson, Department of Emergency Medicine, University of North Carolina School of Medicine; Editor, current and past, *STUDY GUIDE IN EMERGENCY MEDICINE* (all editions since inception).; **floater.**

Blaine C. White, MD, FACEP; *professor emeritus*, emergency medicine, Wayne State University School of Medicine; holder of numerous awards for his contributions to research in emergency medicine, local and national; **floater.**

I am proud of all of you and all you have done.

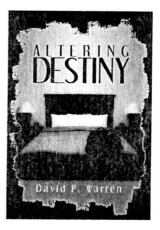
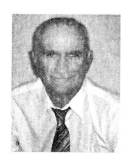

WHISTLING UP THE WIND
THE ADVENTURES OF ANNA MARIE GOLDING
by Kathie Bishop

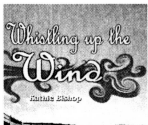
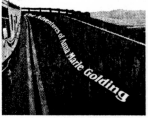

In ancient times, sailors were afraid of women who whistled because they believed that the women would whistle up a storm. Anna Marie Golding has been discouraged from whistling all of her life, but now in her early sixties and widowed for three years, she begins to whistle again. Tired of grieving for her beloved husband, Anna Marie spontaneously buys a Southwind motor home. She sets out for the journey of her life with her faithful pug companion in spite of her family's disgust with her purchase. Along the way, a number of others join her including Christa, a runaway pregnant teenager, and Granny Rose who stows aboard. This is a story of learning to live again after great loss and the love and friendship that develops between these three women. It is also a story of women across the ages, demonstrating their strengths and connections to their ancient pasts.

Paperback, 299pages
6″ x 9″
ISBN 1-4241-9715-5

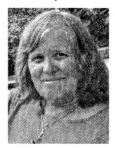

About the author:

Kathleen M. Bishop has a PhD in gerontology. Currently she is the aging consultant for The Arc, Oneida/Lewis Chapter and directs the program on aging and developmental disabilities at the University of Rochester. She has two adult children and lives in upstate New York and Florida with her husband Ron.

WHEN DESTINIES COLLIDE
by Maurice H. Unger

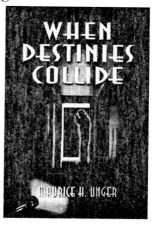

Hurricane Diane, a monster storm, has targeted Virginia Beach, Virginia, as her stepping stone onto the U.S. mainland. Jackie Randolph and her family are unable to evacuate from the resort city before the storm hits. Not only do they experience the harrowing onslaught of this mighty tempest, but they must fight for their lives against a gang of drug traffickers who break into their home at the height of the storm. In a deadly confrontation, Jackie and her father kill two members of the gang, one the brother of the gang leader, Carlos Suarez. Before departing the bloody scene, Carlos swears revenge. Four years later, Carlos exacts a terrible reprisal against the Randolph family, leaving Jackie and her two brothers to pick up the shattered pieces of their lives. An

Paperback, 305 pages
6" x 9"
ISBN 1-4137-7604-3

unsuccessful police investigation causes the beautiful and resourceful Jackie to take the initiative. Will her quest end with an eye for an eye? Deception and intrigue are Jackie's companions as she commences her journey, and at the end, she understands all too well that When Destinies Collide, fate will be the hunter.

About the author:

Born in Alabama and raised in Maryland, Maurice (Maury) is a graduate of the University of the South (Sewanee). He served in the U.S. Navy as a

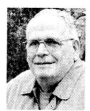

naval flight officer with tours of duty that included operations in Antarctica and flying the A-6E Intruder from the decks of numerous aircraft carriers. Upon retiring from the Navy, he worked in the fields of aviation logistics support and information technology management. He and his wife, Eleanor, reside in Virginia Beach, Virginia. They have two grown sons. This is his first novel.

INSPIRATIONAL CHRISTIAN SPIRITUAL LIVING
by Antonio Cardona

You have picked up a book that will make a difference in your life. Beyond just hearing or reading the Bible, to grow spiritually you need to have the ability to create in your life a better, deeper walk with Christ that jump-starts and moves you closer to the spiritual dimensions intended in the Bible. This is the book that does that. I only suggest what I hope is a deeper understanding of the Jesus parables, sayings, and interesting happenstance stories that can help us live more spiritual lives. Remember, we are only passing through on our way to our real destination!

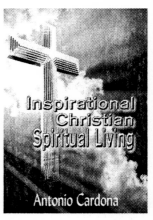

Paperback, 158 pages
5.5" x 8.5"
ISBN 1-60563-917-6

About the author:

Antonio Cardona trains government professionals for his daytime job. He writes and teaches college courses at various New Jersey-based colleges, including Somerset Christian College. He is also involved in professional career counseling and diversity/race relations programming. He holds a master's degree from the Executive Masters in Public Administration Program at Rutgers University and another graduate degree in counseling from the College of New Jersey (formally Trenton State College). He earned dual undergraduate degrees in psychology and religion from Mount Union College. He has served as a counselor and minister in Ohio and Puerto Rico. He lives in New Jersey with Rosa, Teresa, and Daniel. He is a native Spanish speaker

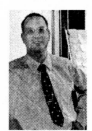